Tropical Medicine

EIGHTH EDITION, REVISED AND EXPANDED

INTERNATIONAL HUMANITARIAN AFFAIRS

Kevin M. Cahill, M.D., series editor

Tropical Medicine

A Clinical Text

EIGHTH EDITION, REVISED AND EXPANDED

KEVIN M. CAHILL, M.D.

FORDHAM UNIVERSITY PRESS
New York   2011

Previous editions:

Cahill KM, 1964. *Tropical Diseases in Temperate Climates*. 225 pp. Lippincott, Philadelphia

Cahill KM, 1976. *Tropical Diseases: A Handbook for Practitioners*. 198 pp. Octopus Press, London

Cahill KM, 1978. *Tropical Diseases: A Handbook for Practitioners*. 225 pp. Technomic, New York

Cahill KM and O'Brien W, 1989. *Tropical Medicine: A Clinical Text*. 261 pp. Anniversary Press, Dublin

Cahill KM and O'Brien W, 1990. *Tropical Medicine: A Clinical Text*. 250 pp. Heinemann UK, U.S., Australia, India and Worldwide Edition

Cahill KM and O'Brien W, 1991. *Medicine Tropicale: Precis Clinique*. 228 pp. Euro-Edition. Brussels

Cahill KM and Gilles HM, 2001. *Tropical Medicine: A Clinical Text*. 260 pp. Center for International Health and Cooperation and The Royal College of Surgeons in Ireland

Cahill, KM and Gilles HM, 2005. *Tropical Medicine: A Clinical Text*. 280 pp. Center for International Health and Cooperation and The Royal College of Surgeons in Ireland; distributed by Fordham University Press

Cover photograph by the author: A mother picking lice (from the hair of her daughter) during a typhus epidemic, Ethiopia, 1964.

The entire International Humanitarian Book Series is available in digital form.

Library of Congress Cataloging-in-Publication Data

Cahill, Kevin M.
   Tropical medicine : a clinical text / Kevin M. Cahill.—8th ed.
     p. ; cm.— (International humanitarian affairs)
   Includes bibliographical references and index.
   Summary: "The history of tropical medicine is as dramatic as the story of mankind—with its own myths and legends, with tales of epidemics destroying whole civilizations; and, still today, with silent stealth, these diseases claim more lives than all the current wars combined. Having had the privilege of working throughout Africa, Asia, and Latin America, as well as in the great medical centers of Europe and the United States, the author presents the essential details for understanding pathogenesis, clinical manifestations, therapy, and prevention of the major tropical diseases. The text, now in its [eighth] edition, has been used for a half-century by medical students, practicing physicians, and public health workers around the world. This fascinating book should also be of interest to a broad, nonmedical readership interested in world affairs. All royalties from the sale of this book go to the training of humanitarian workers"—Provided by publisher.
   ISBN 978-0-8232-4060-9 (cloth : alk. paper)
   ISBN 978-0-8232-4061-6 (paper : alk. paper)
   1. Tropical medicine.   I. Title.   II. Series: International humanitarian affairs (Unnumbered)
[DNLM: 1. Tropical Medicine. WC 680]
RC961.C22   2011
616.9'883—dc23

                       2011021023

Printed in the United States of America
13 12 11 5 4 3 2 1
Eighth edition

For Herself

Contents

Acknowledgments

This book has its origins in a lecture given in 1961 at Bellevue Hospital in New York City. Since I was fortunate to have had a medical elective for a period in Calcutta, India, I was asked to discuss a patient with a tropical disease. My talk included a history of the disease, the usual—and unusual—clinical signs and symptoms, as well as the diagnostic, therapeutic, and public health lessons that could be learned from the individual patient's illness. In the audience was Dr. William Hammond, the distinguished editor-in-chief of *The New York State Journal of Medicine*. He invited me to write a series of articles on "exotic diseases," using the format of my lecture as a template. Thus began the first edition of this book. Some 20 chapters were published, first in a journal, as often were nineteenth-century novels, and then collected into book form.

This text has since been in constant use around the world through seven earlier editions and various translations. It is now issued in its fiftieth year as a revised and expanded Jubilee contribution. In the Old Testament (Leviticus 25), a jubilee is a cause for great celebration: a time to return to one's birthplace or family home, and to express joy with trumpet blasts or, as the name implies, with a ram's horn. There is a personal satisfaction in realizing how much of the original text, particularly the historical notes and clinical descriptions, as well as the photographs of this book, has remained remarkably unchanged. Most of the revisions over the past half-century concerned advances in diagnostic techniques, in drugs used in treatment, and on refinements in our understanding from research on the pathogenesis of infections.

In several earlier editions, I listed dear friends and colleagues as co-authors. Professors William O'Brien and Herbert Gilles taught with me at The Royal College of Surgeons in Ireland (RCSI). Even at that time, neither felt their contributions warranted equal status on the title page because the great bulk of the text was based on my original writings and revisions. Therefore, for this Jubilee Edition, I have accepted their views, and assume full responsibility for this text. In earlier editions, I acknowledged the assistance of other friends and colleagues who kindly reviewed various chapters, provided some visuals, and helped design the text.

As with recent editions, donors to the Tropical Disease Center of Lenox Hill Hospital in New York supported the preparation of this text. It was typed—and re-typed—by Jenna Felz of the staff of The Institute of International Humanitarian Affairs (IIHA) at Fordham University in New York. She also assisted, with exceptional generosity, in every aspect of the editing process. Drs. Alex and Chris Van Tulleken re-read the entire manuscript, offering fresh professional eyes on the work. Mr. Denis Cahill shared in the final copy editing. I express my thanks to Mr. Michael Dowling, CEO of the North Shore–LIJ Medical System, for his enthusiastic support for this edition. Mr. Fredric Nachbaur and the staff of Fordham University Press cooperated professionally and graciously throughout the production of this Jubilee text.

This book is part of the International Humanitarian Affairs Series of Fordham University's IIHA. It provides, along with the *Basics of Humanitarian Missions*, *Emergency Relief Operations*, and other volumes listed at the end of this book, essential practical advice for dealing with the complex problems that almost inevitably follow man-made and natural disasters. These humanitarian crises, more often than not, occur in the less-developed, highly vulnerable nations of the tropics. Statistics on the incidence of disease and the dosages of medications obviously change over time. Most of the data presented in this text reflect figures published in 2010 and are drawn from WHO and other websites cited on page 288.

The dedication in the first edition of this book was "For Herself." This Irish phrase indicates a major influence in a person's life. "Herself" was Kathryn Cahill, my wife and companion of almost 44 years. I submit this work once again in memory of a truly remarkable woman.

Introduction

Knowledge of clinical tropical medicine is essential for every modern physician. The diseases of warm climates are no longer restricted by geographic boundaries because the scope and speed of air travel and flows of ideas and people have destroyed the barriers of time and space, and the massive increase in international migration in the past half century makes us all part of a global community.

The detection of tropical illnesses is utterly dependent on an awareness of their very existence, and on understanding their pathogenesis, signs, and symptoms. These fundamental facts are rarely taught in any depth in Western medical schools, and the diseases considered in this book—the greatest cripplers and killers of the world—rate only passing attention in most academic curricula in temperate climates.

In some European nations, though, there has been a traditional interest in the diseases of the tropics, an interest developed during the colonial period. In these countries there are still major schools (and hospitals) specializing in tropical medicine. Financial support for these institutions has, however, waned in recent decades as the pressures to treat and investigate domestic ailments steadily escalate. In the United States, an appreciation of tropical medicine has always been far less than in Europe.

There are no American schools or hospitals specializing in this discipline, and only a minuscule percentage of our national research budget is allocated to these major albeit neglected diseases. The economic realities of prolonged postgraduate training in the tropics, and the patterns of insurance payments make it difficult to sustain a cadre of experts in tropical medicine. Almost all those whom I have trained, for example, gravitated toward gastroenterology, where colonoscopies and endoscopies are procedures reimbursed at levels far in excess of what is provided to tropicalists.

The quality of laboratory diagnosis in developed countries has also fallen over recent decades. For example, the approach of using wet mount analysis to detect intestinal protozoa is an almost lost art; no longer is the characteristic motility of an ameba able to be detected in specimens sent in preservatives to unknown technicians in distant laboratories. A 2010 study in New York City checked known specimens submitted to a major university hospital laboratory and to the largest commercial medical laboratory in the area. The hospital missed 50%, and the commercial diagnostic inaccuracy rate was 70%.

Learning tropical medicine should not consist of merely memorizing parasitological and microbiological details. A clinical discipline depends on observations, experience, and judgment. My approach in this text is based on the realization that most medical students wish to become practitioners, and that most graduate physicians want the necessary basic information that will allow them to properly care for patients. In tropical medicine, as in other specialties, clinical tools must be learned and constantly refined. I hope that the excitement, wonder, and satisfaction that I have found in the diagnostic and therapeutic challenges of tropical medicine are reflected in these pages, for that surely is my intention.

Based on centuries of clinical contributions, The Royal College of Surgeons of Ireland (RCSI) holds a distinguished position in the history of modern medicine. Today, it is the most international medical school in the Western world. Undergraduate medical students from 35 nations mix with hundreds of graduate doctors who also come from around the world to seek specialty training and certification. The RCSI now has branch medical schools in Malaysia and Bahrain. During my 36-year tenure as Chairman of the Department of Tropical Medicine at RCSI, I taught more than 4,000 medical students using earlier editions of this textbook.

The text is also a product of The Tropical Disease Center of Lenox Hill Hospital. This Center, part of the North Shore–LIJ Medical System, has served thousands of ill and indigent patients, missionaries of all denominations, and United Nations personnel. Finally, the book reflects the efforts of The Center for International Humanitarian Cooperation (CIHC) to alleviate suffering, particularly in war-torn areas, where the breakdown of health services, and the resultant spread of epidemic diseases, usually cause greater morbidity and mortality than gunfire. The CIHC's academic arm for the training of humanitarian workers is the Institute of International Humanitarian Affairs at Fordham University in New York.

Malaria

In the vast underdeveloped areas of the tropics—where the majority of the world's population struggle to exist, and which, in this jet age, have become the playgrounds of tourists, the arenas of diplomatic conflicts, and the reservoirs for expanding business cartels—malaria rules. No other disease so decimates the childhood population, so enfeebles and destroys adults, or serves so well as a reflection of the public health status of an area. By the end of the first decade of the twenty-first century, international health organizations still reported approximately 250 million cases of malaria and nearly 1 million resulting deaths annually, mostly among children living in Africa. In parts of Africa, the disease accounts for 20% of all childhood deaths.

Today, malaria is, once again, a major clinical challenge in the temperate climates, as well, because of the enormous increase in travel to malarious areas combined with a failure on the part of tourists to adhere scrupulously to prophylactic antimalarial regimens. There is, at the time of this writing, no effective vaccine against malaria. The present situation represents one of the great disappointments in modern medicine.

Malaria remains the great tropical disease. Despite the facts that ancient man recognized swamp fevers (malaria), and that more than a century has passed since Ronald Ross demonstrated the transmission of malaria by the female *Anopheline* mosquito, the worldwide risk of infection remains. Possibly the most telling example of the present plight is our humbling return to quinine. More than 300 years ago—long before the parasitology or epidemiology of the disease were known—*Cinchona* alkaloids, in the form of "Jesuit's bark" from "fever trees" growing on the slopes of the Peruvian Andes, were introduced as an effective treatment. Now, despite all the pharmacologic wonders of the twenty-first century, we are grateful that old-fashioned quinine is available. When widespread resistance to this drug develops, and it has already raised its head in southeast Asia, we shall have even more problems dealing with malaria. Fortunately the artemisinin compounds, also derived from an herb, *Artemisia annua*, which has been used as an herbal medicine for more than 2,000 years, now allow us some added breathing space.

In the 1950s, many experts believed that malaria could be eradicated by a combination of aggressive public health programs aimed at destroying the *Anopheline* mosquito vector while simultaneously eliminating the *Plasmodium* parasite reservoir in humans with new synthetic compounds. Neither plan worked well; in many malarious areas, basic health services barely existed, and vast eradication schemes soon fell victim to ineptness as well as to political and military differences that made necessary regional efforts impossible. More significant was the worldwide emergence of parasite strains resistant to drugs as well as mosquitoes increasingly unaffected by potent insecticides.

Even advances in technology—such as the availability of blood banks and transfusions—and changes in societal practices—such as the explosion in intravenous drug abuse—have contributed to the spread of malaria, especially in the more affluent parts of the world. In Europe, the United States, Australia, and most of the former Soviet Union, where endemic malaria had been eradicated, the growth of rapid and relatively cheap air travel has been accompanied by a sharp increase in imported malaria, and airport outbreaks have become a new phenomenon in the Western world. Physicians everywhere must be familiar with the clinical and therapeutic aspects of malaria because there is no other disease that can pass so rapidly from a mild illness, the treatment of which is relatively simple, to a catastrophic state in which the outlook is virtually hopeless. Failure to consider malaria in differential diagnosis, or the inability to recognize parasites in a blood smear, can be a fatal error.

The Parasite

Four species of the genus *Plasmodium* commonly cause disease in human beings. These are *P. vivax* (benign tertian), *P. ovale* (ovale tertian), *P. malariae* (quartan), and *P. falciparum* (malignant tertian). The life cycles of these four malarial parasites are broadly similar, with sexual development (sporogony) occurring in appropriate *Anopheline* mosquito hosts, and asexual maturation (schizogony) occurring in man.

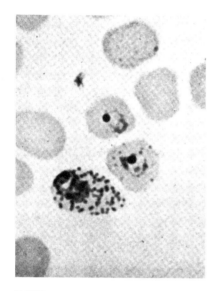

FIGURE 1:

(A) *P. vivax* ameboid trophozoites and a presegmenting schizont. Note prominent Schuffner's dots.

FIGURE 1:

(B) Mixed infection with *P. vivax* and *P. falciparum*.

During the act of biting an infected person, *Anopheles* mosquitoes may ingest male and female gametocytes. The male exflagellates in the insect gut and fertilizes a female parasite. The resulting oocyst then enlarges in the stomach wall of the mosquito for 7 to 20 days before rupturing into the body cavity, releasing thousands of sporozoites. Those that lodge in the salivary glands may be injected into a new victim when the mosquito bites.

Sporozoites remain in the human blood stream for less than an hour. A few of them penetrate parenchymal cells of the liver and undergo pre-erythrocytic schizogony. When the hepatic schizont ruptures 5 to 16 days later (see Table 1), merozoites are liberated into the blood stream.

The pre-erythrocytic merozoites then enter red blood cells, enlarge from a ring form to a mature trophozoite and finally a schizont, which

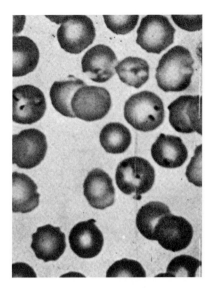

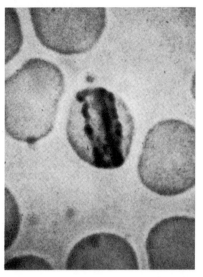

FIGURE 1:
(C) Early *P. falciparum trophozoites*. Note multiple infections and appliqué forms.

FIGURE 1:
(D) *P. malariae*, "band" form trophozoite.

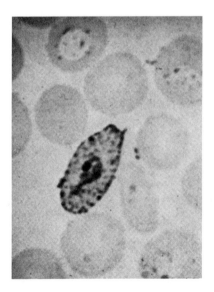

FIGURE 1:
(E) Ameboid *P. ovale* trophozoite.

again may rupture, liberating merozoites that invade other red blood cells. This cycle of development takes 48 hours (tertian malaria) to 72 hours (quartan malaria). The severity of the pathological changes and manifestations is directly proportional to the percentage of cells parasitized. Because *P. vivax* and *P. ovale* preferentially attack reticulocytes, and *P. malariae* attacks only aging red cells, less than 2% of erythrocytes are affected. However, *P. falciparum* may invade erythrocytes of all ages, and severe degrees of parasitemia are not uncommon. A few trophozoites do not develop into schizonts, but rather into male and female gametocytes that may be ingested by mosquitoes to renew the sexual cycle.

In *P. vivax* and *P. ovale*, infections some of the sporozoites may, on entering the liver cells, remain in a dormant phase (hypnozoites). These hypnozoites are genetically programmed to commence active division after a predetermined interval, depending on the particular strain of the parasite, thus causing long incubation periods or the relapses characteristic of these infections.

Pathology

The pathological changes are related to the development of asexual parasites in the blood. Rupture of the red cells and liberation of merozoites into the plasma is attended by a bout of fever; when the development of the parasites are in step, as in established infections, these bouts of fever occur at regular intervals. If sufficient red cells are destroyed, anemia with hyperbilirubinemia can develop, but these effects are usually only significant in *P. falciparum* malaria. The debris from red cell destruction is taken up by reticuloendothelial cells, especially in the spleen and liver, and these organs enlarge. Among this debris is the pigment hemozoin, the byproduct of hemoglobin digestion by the parasite, and this may be seen as brown granules in reticuloendothelial cells and white blood cells. Thrombocytopenia is common.

In *P. falciparum* malaria, there is usually a higher degree of parasitemia, and the maturation of these parasites takes place almost exclusively in the vascular beds of internal organs rather than in the peripheral blood stream. During the maturation process, protrusions of the parasitized cell membrane develop and attach to capillary and

Table 1. Life cycle and morphological characteristics of *plasmodium* parasites causing malaria in human beings

Plasmodium species	Pre-erythrocytic period (days)	Cycle time (hours)	Persistence in man (years)	Characteristics of parasitized red cells
P. vivax	8	48	5	Enlarged; Schuffner's dots 12 to 24 merozoites
P. falciparum	5	48	2	Not enlarged; Maurer's clefts; accole and appliqué forms; multiple in one red blood cell — 12 to 24 merozoites; black pigments prominent; schizonts rare in peripheral blood; crescent-shaped gametocytes
P. malariae	16	72	40	Not enlarged; Ziemann's dots; band forms — 6 to 12 merozoites; daisy-head form of schizonts
P. ovale	9	48	5	Enlarged — 6 to 12 merozoites; fimbriated ends

venous endothelium. This is best demonstrated in the brain, where focal aggregations of parasitized erythrocytes impede cerebral blood flow, resulting in hypoxia and impairment of glucose metabolism. The pathogenesis of cerebral malaria is complex, but the basis is a selective adhesion of parasitized cells to cerebral vascular endothelium, brought about by a variety of changes in infected erythrocytes, with a number of possible receptors responsible. Anemia may be severe due to hemolysis and dyshemopoesis, and jaundice may be deep. Another common pathophysiologic cascade begins with dehydration and hyponatremia precipitating peripheral vascular collapse, prerenal uremia, and finally, acute renal failure with tubular necrosis.

Repeated malarial infections induce a slowly increasing degree of immunity, which is partial where transmission is irregular, but almost complete in individuals living in hyperendemic regions where transmission occurs all the year round. This immunity is associated with high plasma levels of IgG antibodies that traverse the placenta, protecting the fetus from congenital malaria and also giving the infant a considerable degree of passive immunity during the first 3 to 6 months of life. Thereafter, the child may be exposed to recurring attacks of malaria, which peak at 2 to 5 years and are accompanied by hepatosplenomegaly. If the child survives, an increasing degree of immunity develops after the age of 4 to 5 years. Indirect consequences of malaria include a high prevalence of congenital red cell disorders and Burkitt's lymphoma.

Clinical Features

Although infection is usually acquired following a mosquito bite, it may also be transmitted through the use of contaminated blood, needles, and syringes, as well as following organ transplants. Congenital malaria also occurs but is rare in regions of stable malaria. The popular conception of a malarial attack is most commonly seen in *P. vivax* infection. The incubation period is usually 8 to 10 days, but may be some months. There is an abrupt onset with chills, shivering, or a frank rigor, usually about midday or in the early afternoon. This is the "cold stage," lasting an hour, during which the temperature rises rapidly. This is followed by the "hot stage," lasting 4 to 6 hours, during which there is high

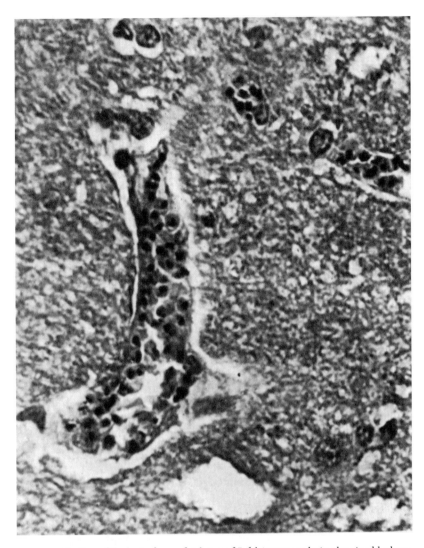

FIGURE 2: Section of the brain from a fatal case of *P. falciparum* malaria, showing blockage of capillaries with pigment and parasites.

fever; headache; malaise; and not uncommonly, abdominal pain, vomiting, thirst, and polyuria. This in turn is followed by a "sweating stage" of 1 to 2 hours, during which the temperature falls back to normal, and the symptoms clear.

In primary attacks, bouts of fever may occur daily for the first few days before the fever settles into the characteristic tertian pattern. As bouts continue, the spleen becomes palpable, and herpes labialis may appear. In children, the manifestations are often atypical and may be alarming. Paroxysms of fever are less common, while headache, nausea, vomiting, abdominal pain, diarrhea, a sustained fever, and convulsions make up a much less characteristic clinical picture. In anemic children with a high proportion of reticulocytes, the illness may be particularly severe, and repeated attacks may lead to malarial cachexia and chronic hepatosplenomegaly. *P. vivax* malaria is rarely fatal; in a major epidemic in Sri Lanka, with 537,705 reported cases, there was not a single death. The most important potentially fatal complication is rupture of the spleen.

The red cell receptor for *P. vivax* is associated with the Duffy blood group, and because many Africans are Duffy blood group–negative, *P. vivax* malaria is rare in sub-Saharan Africa, where it is replaced by *P. ovale* malaria. The clinical features are indistinguishable from those of P. *vivax* malaria.

The incubation period of *P. malariae*, which tends to have a similar geographic distribution to *P. falciparum* infection, can vary from 16 to as long as 28 days. The attacks of fever are similar to those seen in *P. vivax* malaria, but occur every 72 hours instead of 48 hours. If untreated, a low parasitemia may persist for many years causing a recrudescent malaria, frequently associated with some temporary decline or loss of immunity. The most serious complication of P. *malariae* infection is an immune complex type of glomerular nephritis affecting children, with a peak incidence at 5 to 7 years of age. Massive nonselective proteinuria results in hypoalbuminemia and gross edema. This condition does not improve with antimalarial treatment, and only a small proportion of such children respond to steroid or immunosuppressive therapy.

The incubation period of *P. falciparum* malaria is usually about 5 to 7 days. In contrast to the other types of malaria, the onset is often insidious, and medical care may not be sought for several days. In children, however, the interval between the onset of symptoms and death may be as short as 48 hours. These patients may present with a flu-like illness, with fever, headache, dizziness, malaise, aches, and pains, but shaking chills are often absent. Jaundice, which is not uncommon, may be mistaken for viral hepatitis. Some patients may not experience fever at all. Associated symptoms are variable, but may include nausea, vomiting, and a bronchitic cough. Although diarrhea is often listed as a symptom in older texts, it is, in fact, uncommon, except in children. The fever is irregular, commonly with no tertiary pattern, and splenomegaly is also inconstant.

In *P. falciparium* malaria, unrecognized and untreated patients are liable to present with one or more pernicious manifestations.

Cerebral Malaria

This acute encephalopathy accounts for more than 80% of deaths from malaria. The majority of the dead are children younger than age 5. The syndrome may start with increasing headache, restlessness, or even bizarre behavior. A generalized convulsion is often followed by increasing drowsiness, going on to stupor and coma. Physical examination reveals a symmetric upper-motor neuron lesion with extensor posturing and dysconjugate gaze. There may be papilledema or retinal hemorrhage. A lumbar puncture is essential to exclude meningitis or subarachnoid hemorrhage, but in cerebral malaria, the spinal fluid is usually normal, or at the most, shows only a slight rise in protein or cells.

Acute Renal Failure

Although usually occurring in patients with other manifestations of acute malaria, this dangerous complication may be the presenting feature in an afebrile patient. It is preceded by oliguria and prerenal uremia, leading often to complete anuria with a urine of fixed specific gravity (around 1,010) and rapidly rising blood urea, creatinine, and potassium. It is an uncommon complication in children.

Hypoglycemia

This condition should be suspected in any patient with altered consciousness, convulsions, or an abnormal respiratory pattern. In children and in pregnant women, it is not infrequently a presenting symptom; in adults, and occasionally also in children, it occurs as a result of treatment with intravenous quinine. The classical symptoms of hypo-glycemia may often be absent.

Metabolic Acidosis

Lactic acidosis is the major contributory mechanism. In children, it often presents with respiratory distress. Deep breathing in the absence of chest signs is a good clinical indicator of the presence of acidosis. When associated with severe anemia (Hgb <5 g per ml), resuscitation with rapid transfusion of blood results in marked clinical improvement. In less-anemic children, rapid transfusion of crystalloids results in sharp falls in serum lactate.

Severe Anemia

This is common, but particularly so—and often fatal—in African children or pregnant primiparous women who have previously been immune.

Algid Malaria

This is an acute shock syndrome with vascular collapse. The pulse is rapid and of poor volume or may even be impalpable. There is severe arterial hypotension, and the peripheral blood pressure often cannot be measured. Again, this syndrome may be a presenting feature, may occur during the course of treatment, or be the first evidence of a gram nega-tive septicemia.

Disseminated Intravascular Coagulation

This appears to be less common than has been suggested in the litera-ture. Significant thrombocytopenia is, on the other hand, common and can cause bleeding.

Acute Respiratory Distress Syndrome (Idiopathic Pulmonary Edema)

Pulmonary edema in malaria arises in association with severe acidosis and renal failure. A usually fatal idiopathic pulmonary disorder of uncertain origin, presenting as a respiratory distress syndrome, has also been described. Careful intravenous rehydration is essential if one is to avoid overloading the circulation in severe *P. falciparum* infection.

Hemoglobinuria

Hemoglobinuria with acute renal failure in patients with few, if any, demonstrable parasites in the peripheral blood are the features of blackwater fever. The condition was often associated with quinine therapy, but the causal connection between drug and disorder has never been proved. The condition now appears to be uncommon, but a similar syndrome may occur in patients with malaria and glucose 6 phosphate dehydrogenase (G6PD) deficiency, especially in those treated with primaquine or various sulfa compounds.

Fluid and Electrolyte Disturbances

Patients are often dehydrated on admission, and a variety of fluid and electrolyte abnormalities are common, particularly hyponatremia.

Important differences in the manifestations of severe malaria between adults and children are given in Table 2.

Diagnosis

The most important aspect in the clinical diagnosis of malaria is to have a high index of suspicion, and to develop the habit of always eliciting a travel history. One must always remember that malaria is a great mimic of other diseases. The most common misdiagnoses, with fatal consequences, are influenza, viral hepatitis, meningitis, and viral encephalitis. Confirmation of a clinical diagnosis of malaria classically depends upon finding *Plasmodium* parasites in blood smears. Thick films should be examined for the presence of parasites, and thin films allow for species differentiation.

However, if *P. falciparum* infection is suspected, treatment should proceed without waiting for confirmation. An apparently mild illness can become lethal within a few hours. A dangerous infection may be present in patients with a peripheral parasitemia so sparse as to be

Table 2. Differences between severe malaria in adults and children*

Sign or symptom	Adults	Children
History of cough	Uncommon	Common
Convulsions	Common	Very common
Duration of illness	5 to 7 days	1 to 2 days
Resolution of coma	2 to 4 days	1 to 2 days
Neurological sequelae	<5%	>10%
Jaundice	Common	Uncommon
Pretreatment hypoglycemia	Uncommon	Common
Pulmonary edema	Uncommon	Rare
Renal failure	Common	Uncommon
CSF opening pressure	Usually normal	Usually raised
Respiratory distress (acidosis)	Sometimes	Common
Bleeding/clotting disturbances	Up to 10%	Rare
Abnormality of brain stem reflexes (e.g. oculovestibular, oculocervical)	Rare	More common

*Derived from WHO studies in southeast Asian adults and children, and African children

undetectable by routine methods. This is especially likely when a patient has taken inadequate prophylactic antimalarial drugs or has been treated with antibacterial agents. On the other hand, it must also be realized that an apparent response to antimalarial drugs does not exclude other serious causes of fever such as typhoid. Fewer than 5% of patients with malaria have a leukocytosis, and this should prompt a search for an additional or alternative diagnosis.

Although thick and thin films remain the mainstay of diagnosis worldwide, molecular diagnostic techniques are increasingly available. In developed countries, polymearase chain reaction (PCR) testing provides results that are highly sensitive and specific, though time-consuming and expensive. In developing countries the falling cost of immunochromatographic rapid tests has allowed improved diagnosis in regions and contexts where microscopy in laboratory facilities is often inaccurate. High annual volumes of tests (>2,000 tests/year) should prompt consideration of the cost effectiveness of laboratory construction and operation as a viable alternative to rapid testing.

Treatment

Uncomplicated Malaria

The most important element in treatment is to bring the parasitemia under control as quickly as possible by the administration of rapidly acting schizonticidal drugs. This presents little difficulty except in *P. falciparum* malaria. Standard, very effective, treatment for *P. vivax*, *P. ovale*, and *P. malariae* is with oral chloroquine diphosphate. The adult dose (adult dose given throughout) is 600 mg base, followed in 6 hours by 300 mg, base, and then 300 mg base on each of the next 2 days. For children, the corresponding doses are 10 mg base per kg bw and initially followed by 2 days of 5 mg per kg base dose. Toxic effects are rare and are confined to headache, occasional slight blurring of vision, and in Africans, pruritus. Psychological side effects have been occasionally reported. The drug can be administered to pregnant women. Resistance of *P. vivax* to chloroquine has been reported, but at present, it is limited to a few countries. In areas with chloroquine resistant *P. vivax*, treatment with artemisinin-based combination therapies is recommended.

Chloroquine has no effective action on hypnozoites, so that if a radical cure of *P. vivax* or *P. ovale* infections is sought to prevent relapses, primaquine diphosphate should also be given in a daily dose of 15 mg for 2 to 3 weeks. There is little point in giving primaquine to patients remaining in endemic areas, nor should this drug be given to young children or pregnant women. It is also contraindicated in patients who are G6PD-deficient. The treatment of even uncomplicated *P. falciparum* malaria is more difficult because of widespread resistance to antimalarial drugs and because of the severe complications that are liable to occur. Where parasites are sensitive to chloroquine—as in Central America—that drug remains highly effective, giving a radical cure. There is now widespread resistance throughout Africa, southeast Asia, and Latin America. WHO now recommends using artesunate combination therapy (ACTs) for treatment of all *P. falciparum* malaria. The artemisinin derivative components of the combination must be given for at least 3 days.

Artemether plus lumefantrine, distributed under the trade name Coartem, was the first licensed ACT and is still the most widely used. It is licensed for use in the United States. Coartem is available as tablets containing 20 mg of artemether and 120 mg of lumefantrine. A total of 16 tablets is taken on a specific schedule over 3 days.

If local drug sensitivities are unknown, dihydroaretmisinin plus piperaquine is also an effective ACT option for first-line treatment in almost all regions. Full therapy includes an initial dose of 4 mg per kg per day dihydroartemisinin and 18 mg per kg per day piperaquine for 3 days. This ACT is currently available as a fixed-dose combination with tablets containing 40 mg of dihydroartemisinin and 320 mg of piperaquine.

Other options now recommended for treatment of uncomplicated *P. falciparum* malaria are:

Artesunate plus amodiaquine
Artesunate plus mefloquine
Artesunate plus sulfadoxine-pyrimethamine

There is still substantial regional variation in the efficacy of different ACTs (determined by local resistance to the artemisinin's partner medication), and national guidelines and therapeutic decisions should reflect continuous monitoring of this to ensure use of the appropriate ACT.

Recommended second-line treatments for uncomplicated *P. falciparum* malaria include an alternative ACT, artesunate plus tetracycline or doxycycline or clindamycin for 7 days, and quinine plus tetracycline or doxycycline or clindamycin for 7 days. A new classification of antimalarial drug resistance takes into account both clinical and parasitological resistance as well as the intensity of malaria transmission.

Severe P. falciparum *Malaria*

Severe *P. falciparum* malaria is a medical emergency: Full doses of parenteral antimalarial treatment should be started the first effective antimalarial available immediately after clinical assessment and diagnosis (Guidelines for the Treatment of Malaria, 2nd edition, World Health Organization, 2010).

Intravenous (IV) artesunate should be used in preference to quinine for the treatment of severe *P. falciparum* malaria in adults. This therapy has been shown to significantly reduce the risk of death from severe malaria compared with IV quinine and is associated with a lower risk of hypoglycemia.

Artesunate offers a number of therapeutic advantages over quinine, not requiring rate-controlled infusion or cardiac monitoring.

Treatment for adults is as follows:

Recommended: Artesunate 2.4 mg per kg bw IV or IM given on admission (time = 0), then at 12 h and 24 h, then once daily.

Quinine is an acceptable alternative if parenteral artesunate is not available: quinine 20 mg salt per kg bw on admission (IV infusion or divided IM injection), then 10 mg per kg bw every 8 h; infusion rate should not exceed 5 mg salt per kg bw per hour.

Quinidine is considered more toxic than either artestunate or quinine (commonly causing hypotension and QT prolongation). This drug should be used only in the context of electrocardiographic monitoring and frequent assessment of vital signs and if no other effective parenteral drugs are available.

Treatment for children is as follows. There is currently insufficient evidence to indicate that any one of these parenteral antimalarial medicines is more effective than another:

Artesunate 2.4 mg per kg bw IV or IM given on admission (time = 0), then at 12 h and 24 h, then once daily.

Quinine 20 mg salt per kg bw on admission (IV infusion or divided IM injection), then 10 mg per kg bw every 8 h; infusion rate should not exceed 5 mg salt per kg bw per hour.

Artemether 3.2 mg per kg bw IM given on admission, then 1.6 mg per kg bw per day should be used only if none of the alternatives are available because its absorption may be erratic.

In patients with complicated *P. falciparum* malaria, parenteral antimalarials should be used for a minumum of 24 hours once started. Following initial parenteral treatment, after the patient can tolerate oral therapy, it is essential to provide a complete course of an ACT or quinine plus clindamycin or doxycycline.

There is insufficient information on the safety and efficacy of most antimalarials in *pregnancy*, but current data suggest few adverse effects of ACTs on pregnancy or on the health of the fetus and neonates. Current recommendations for *P. falciparum* malaria in pregnancy are quinine plus clindamycin to be given for 7 days; artesunate plus clindamycin for 7 days is indicated if this treatment fails. Quinine is not contraindicated in severe malaria in pregnancy because the risk of malaria to mother and child far outweigh the risk of quinine.

Evidence on the safety and efficacy of ACTs in *infants and young children* is still limited, but current WHO recommendations are that ACTs should be used as first-line treatment for infants and young children with uncomplicated malaria, avoiding sulfadoxine-pyrimethamine and primaquine in the first few weeks, and tetracyclines in children <8 years of age. With these exceptions, there is no evidence for specific serious toxicity for any of the other currently recommended antimalarial treatments in infancy.

In addition to the drug therapy noted above, patients with cerebral malaria need *complementary management*: They should be nursed on alternate sides, and frequent pharyngeal suction is helpful in keeping the airways clear. If convulsions do develop, they are best controlled by slow IV infusion of diazepam. Lumbar puncture to exclude meningitis should be performed, or coverage with an appropriate antibiotic instituted. It is necessary to carefully monitor urinary output. Oliguria demands the prompt correction of fluid and electrolyte balance, and if necessary, diuretics and an infusion of dopamine. Dialysis is required for acute renal failure. The body temperature should be maintained below 101°F, if necessary by tepid sponging, fanning, and paracetamol. A hemoglobin concentration less than 5 g per 100 ml calls for a transfusion of fresh whole blood given very slowly over 4 hours. A parasitemia of more than 20% is best treated by an exchange transfusion, if facilities are available. The rapid and broad range of action of artesunate or artemether, clearing 95% of parasitemia within a few hours, may render this procedure unnecessary.

Gram negative septicemia requires parenteral antibiotics and correction of hemodynamic disturbances. Quinine is a powerful stimulant of insulin secretion, and patients must be carefully monitored for hypoglycemia, which if it arises, can be treated by a 50% dextrose injection followed by 5% to 10% dextrose infusion. Somastostatin infusion has been used successfully in refractory cases. Hypoglycemia seems to be a particularly serious complication for pregnant women with *P. falciparum* malaria. Pregnant women also will require careful obstetric monitoring, and in late pregnancy, Caesarian section should be considered as it may be life-saving for both mother and child.

Prevention

Preventive measures may be considered under the headings of those used by the community and those conferring a degree of personal protection.

For community protection, the reservoir of infection can best be reduced by the early recognition and prompt adequate treatment of malarial attacks. Efforts at vector control focus on the sites where *Anopheline* larvae develop; collections of standing water can be drained or filled in; stagnant streams can be cleared; and the use of larvicides; such as Temephos (Abate); can be employed. In certain circumstances, the introduction of larviverous fish has proved useful. In urban areas, mosquitoes can usually be best controlled by the use of residual insecticides although, as already noted, resistance to, and toxicity of, these chemicals pose major public health challenges. Pyrethroid impregnated nets have been shown to reduce malaria morbidity and mortality in areas of both high and low transmission. Long-term insecticide-impregnated nets (Olyset: Permanet) are preferable. They retain their effectiveness for several years despite frequent washing of nets.

For individual protection, while the wearing of suitable clothing in the evening, using repellents, mosquito-proofing, and insecticide-impregnated mosquito nets are very important, nonimmune visitors to endemic areas require individual chemoprophylaxis. In regions where there is no chloroquine resistance, chloroquine 300 mg weekly with proguanil 200 mg daily are of proved value, and both drugs can safely be used in pregnancy. Where there is drug resistance, the choice is between mefloquine (250 mg weekly), doxycycline (100 mg daily), or malarone (a combination of atovaquone and proguanil). The risk of side effects of these drugs must be carefully weighed against the risk of acquiring malaria, particularly in the case of short-term visitors. None of the preceding is recommended in the first trimester of pregnancy, and ideally, pregnant women should avoid going to malarious areas in the first trimester or avoid getting pregnant while on prophylaxis. This is a feasible option for short-term visitors, but of course, not for long-term sojourns in the tropics. For this group maximal personal protection is needed together with early diagnosis and prompt treatment. Whatever prophylactic is used, individuals must be warned that protection is never 100%, and that they may still develop malaria. It should also be stressed that they must continue to take their prophylactics for at least 28 days after leaving an endemic area. Malarone is continued for only 7 days. Additional terminal prophylaxis with primaquine may also be necessary for those who have had significant exposure to *P. vivax* infection in Latin America, India, and southeast Asia.

Drug prophylaxis is also advised for certain groups of indigenous people living in endemic areas; these include pregnant women, particularly primiparae; persons with sickle cell disease; and children being treated for malnutrition. Meanwhile, a great deal of effort is on-going to produce a vaccine, and several promising clinical trials are underway. Even if these prove successful, however, it will take years before a vaccine is fully tested and available for general use.

Intermittent preventive therapy in pregnancy (IPTp) given in the second and third trimester has been shown to be effective in reducing placental parasitemia, improving birth weight, and reducing severe maternal anemia. Similarly intermittent preventive therapy for malaria in infants (IPTi) reduces malaria attacks and anemia in the first year of life. In this strategy, infants receive an appropriate antimalarial drug 3 times during the first year of life, regardless of whether they have malaria, at the time of routine infant immunization. The antimalarial drug chosen would depend on the resistance situation.

Hyperactive Malarial Splenomegaly

Hyperactive malarial splenomegaly, or the tropical splenomegaly syndrome, or big spleen disease, is characterized by splenomegaly, often massive, and lymphocytic infiltration of the hepatic sinusoids. It is probably due to an abnormal immunological response to repeated malarial infection; it is one of the most common causes of gross spleno-megaly in sub-Saharan Africa and Papua New Guinea.

Pathology

The spleen may weigh more than 4,000 g. Widely dilated sinuses are lined by swollen reticulum cells exhibiting marked erythrohagocytosis but no malarial pigment. The liver is also often enlarged with dilated sinuses containing lymphocytes. Malarial parasites are rarely found, but serum examination reveals a high IgM concentration and a raised titer of malarial antibodies. Hypersplenism can cause a moderate anemia, leukopenia, and thrombocytopenia.

Clinical Features

There is a gradual onset of fatigue that can progress to an incapacitating weakness. Left upper-quadrant pain is common, and many patients can palpate a tumor mass. Pregnant women may suffer attacks of acute hemolysis requiring urgent treatment. Physical examination reveals gross splenomegaly in an afebrile patient, evidence of hypervolemia, and moderate anemia. The liver is also often enlarged.

Diagnosis

Other causes of gross splenomegaly in endemic areas must first be excluded. Confirmatory evidence for this syndrome is given by finding a high level of serum IgM, raised titers of malarial antibody, and on liver biopsy, lymphocytic infiltration of hepatic sinuses.

Treatment

Patients respond well to treatment with proguanil 200 mg daily. After 6 to 12 months, the spleen will have retracted and symptoms cleared, but it is essential that treatment continue indefinitely to prevent relapse. Splenectomy is an alternative treatment but should not be attempted in patients who will continue to reside in the tropics.

Babesiosis

Babesiae are intraerythrocytic ring- and rod-shaped bodies of the genus *Piroplasma*; they closely resemble malarial parasites but contain no pigment. They multiply within the red cell into a tetrad resembling a Maltese cross. There are several species that can parasitize cattle, dogs, rodents, and other animals, and are transmitted between these animals by *Ixodes* ticks. Two species, *Babesia bovis* and *B. microti*, may also infect man.

Since 1968, *B. microti* infection has been endemic in the northeast United States, especially along the coast of New England and New York. The main reservoir hosts for *B. microti* are deer mice and meadow voles. The vector is the northern deer tick, *Ixodes dammini*. During its larval and nymph stages, the tick feeds primarily on rodents but has also been found on domestic animals and man. During its adult life, the tick's main host is the white-tailed deer. It is probably the nymphal instar that is responsible for transmission of the infection to man.

Patients may or may not give a history of a tick bite, but all patients, except those who have acquired the infection from a blood transfusion, will have been exposed to ticks. Infection may remain asymptomatic, or there may be a gradual onset of anorexia, fatigue, and sweating with generalized myalgia. Later, there may be high fever with rigors, but the fever shows no periodicity. In one-third of patients with acute babesiosis, there is a mild splenomegaly and, occasionally, mild hepatic enlargement.

There is a varying degree of hemolytic anemia. *B. microti* in blood films closely resemble the small rings of *P. falciparum* malaria. The parasites may also be demonstrated following injection of the patient's blood into splenectomized hamsters. Serum antibody to *B. microti* can commonly be demonstrated by indirect immunofluorescence over the subsequent 2 to 6 months.

Chloroquine, quinine, and pyrimethamine have little or no curative effect. Most patients recover spontaneously but sometimes only after an illness that may last several months. The current treatment of choice is a combination of clindamycin and quinine sulfate. Should this infection occur in a splenectomized person, the illness may be much more severe, and exchange transfusion may be life-saving. Concomitant Lyme disease and erlichiosis, both transmitted by the same *Ixodid* ticks, occurs.

Babesia bovis is a common parasite of cattle in Europe. The illness in cattle is known as Redwater Fever and is transmitted by hard ticks. Only 7 human infections have been reported, all in splenectomized persons, and 5 of the patients died.

The Trypanosomatidae

.

Tens of thousands of arable African acres lie fallow today because of trypanosomiasis. In tropical areas where food shortage and malnutrition causes so much infant mortality and adult morbidity, such waste of land is disastrous. For the visitor from a temperate climate, the persistence of sleeping-sickness zones may curtail travel plans and even pose a lethal threat for those on safari. In South America and Central America, trypanosomal infections kill young and old alike. As immigration from the poor rural areas of Latin America expands, the threat of transmission through blood transfusion in the cities increases.

In temperate climates, the chronic manifestations of Chagas' disease are presenting diagnostic challenges with increasing frequency. Throughout wide areas of Latin America, Africa, and the Near and the Far East, the dermatological lesions caused by *Leishmania*, a closely related genus of parasites, are deforming thousands each year, and visceral infection with this organism still claims its annual toll. Trypanosomal and leishmanial diseases of man differ widely in their geographic distribution, vectors, pathology, clinical manifestations, prognosis, and response to treatment. Nonetheless, all these diseases have certain features in common because the etiological parasites are all members of the family *Trypanosomatidae*. They are all protozoa, and each of them may assume several or all four developmental forms:

The amastigote (leishmanial form) is an oval organism 2 to 5 microns in diameter. It is found in the tissues of patients with all types of leishmaniasis and the American form of trypanosomiasis. The organism has neither an external flagellum nor an undulating membrane.

The promastigote (leptomonad form) is the infective form found in insect vectors, cultures of leishmania, and as a transitional stage in human beings with American trypanosomiasis. This form is characterized by an elongated shape 10 to 15 micrometers in length, a free flagellum, no undulating membrane, and a kinetoplast far anterior to the nucleus.

The epimastigote (crithidial form) has a kinetoplast just anterior to the nucleus and also a free flagellum, but has no undulating membrane. It is found on culture and in the insect vectors of all human trypanosomal infections.

The trypanomastigote (trypanosome form) is a motile flagellate form that can be found in the blood, lymphatic tissue, and cerebrospinal fluid of infected animal hosts, including man. In blood films of patients with American trypanosomiasis, the monomorphic parasite assumes a "C" or a "U" shape and has a prominent posterior kinetoplast. In African infections, the parasite is polymorphic and may be short and stumpy, or long and thin.

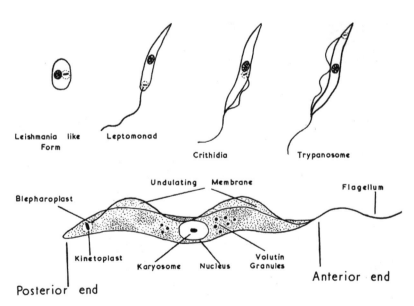

FIGURE 3: Developmental forms of the family Trypanosomatidae.

Trypanosomiases

African Trypanosomiasis

In Africa, two trypanosomes cause human disease. West African sleeping sickness is caused by *Trypanosoma brucei gambiense*, and East African sleeping sickness is caused by by *Trypanosoma brucei rhodesiense*. The insect vectors of both diseases are tsetse flies; the West African type is transmitted by riverine flies of the *Glossina palpalis* group, while the East African variety is spread by the *Glossina morsitans* group, which inhabits woodland, bush, and thicket.

Man is probably the main reservoir of *T. gambiense*, whereas wild game are the predominant hosts of *T. rhodesiense*. Therefore, the habits of the parasites and their vectors determine the epidemiology of human disease. West African trypanosomiasis poses a severe threat to large numbers of people who use rivers for washing, drinking, fishing, or transportation. The East African disease primarily affects those who live in or enter the game-inhabited woodland or bush. The presence of an infection can rapidly depopulate a river valley, and the risk of disease prevents vast fertile areas from being cultivated.

Sleeping sickness once decimated Africa; in the early years of the twentieth century, more than one million deaths occurred in the Congo alone, and in one outbreak around Lake Victoria, 200,000 of a total population of 300,000 died within 8 years. Unfortunately, many of the regional sleeping-sickness control measures have become the victims of other national priorities; military expenditures, corruption, and complacency have eroded the public health foundations in many new African nations, and trypanosomiasis has now resurfaced as a major threat. Recent outbreaks have occurred in Central and East African countries.

Pathology

The usual mode of infection is through the injection of metacyclic infective trypanosomes beneath the dermis by the *Glossina* fly. Congenital transmission and infection by needle-prick accidents in the laboratory are also described. At the site of inoculation, an indurated, erythematous "chancre" may form in which the metacyclic form of the parasite multiplies over a period of 2 to 3 weeks before entering the

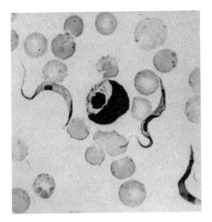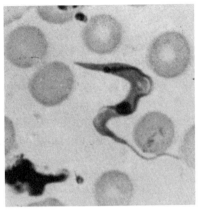

FIGURE 4: *Trypanosoma gambiense* in the peripheral blood of a patient with West African sleeping sickness.

circulation. There is diffuse reticuloendothelial proliferation, with lymphadenopathy prominent, particularly in the Gambian infection. Trypanosomes are by no means confined to the blood or lymphatics. Cellular degeneration with infiltration of monocytes, lymphocytes, large lymphoid cells, and plasma cells may be seen in various tissues although the pathogenesis of these lesions remains unclear. Myocarditis is described in *T. rhodesiense* infection.

The parasites excite vigorous but ineffective humoral immune reaction. The infecting trypanosomes have heterogeneous glycoprotein coats. As one antigen becomes predominant and is destroyed, it is replaced by another variant, and this process continues indefinitely. The predominant antibodies belong to the IgM immunoglobulin type.

After a variable time, quite short in *T. rhodesiense* infection but sometimes years with *T. gambiense*, trypanosomes establish themselves in the central nervous system. The meninges become covered with a fibrinous exudate, and the gyri may be flattened as a result of diffuse cerebral edema. In the thickened pia arachnoid, mononuclear infiltration around small vessels produces perivascular cuffing, and free trypanosomes may be found in brain tissue. Large morular cells of Mott, the cytoplasm of which consists of a number of clear spherules containing IgM, are pathognomonic. Cerebrospinal fluid protein and cells are increased. Death most commonly is caused by intercurrent infection.

Clinical Features

In a minority of patients, a painful, circumscribed, rubbery, indurated, dusky red lesion, 2 to 5 cm across, develops at the site of the tsetse bite. It may resemble a blind boil with a waxy center, and is hot to touch, but subsides spontaneously within 2 to 3 weeks. Systemic infection is manifest by an irregular relapsing fever with concomitant tachycardia, which persists during apyrexial intervals. With the fever, there is headache, often severe; weakness; fatigue; malaise; excessive sweating at night; loss of appetite and weight; diffuse aches and pains; and sometimes generalized itching. In light-skinned persons, a circinate, erythematous rash may be seen.

Periorbital edema, giving the face a swollen, sullen, rather sad expression, is common. There may be swelling of the hands and feet. An important sign, if present, is enlargement of lymph nodes, particularly in the posterior cervical chain (Winterbottom's sign); the spleen may also be palpable. In *T. gambiense* infection, the bouts of fever gradually become less severe and less frequent. In *T. rhodesiense* infection, on the other hand, they often persist, the patient's condition progressively deteriorating with serous effusions, cardiac involvement, intercurrent infections, and acute encephalopathy leading rapidly to death.

The first sign of central nervous system involvement is often a change of mood apparent only to the patient's close associates. A normally cheerful meticulous person may become indifferent, disinclined to any effort, careless in his appearance, withdrawn, morose, and quarrelsome. There may be insomnia with mood swings and antisocial behavior, quite out of keeping with the individual's previous character, resulting in involvement with the police or commitment to a mental institution.

Other symptoms include headache, daytime somnolence, loss of libido or impotence, amenorrhea, and intense pruritus leading to excoriation of the skin. A curious finding, known as "Kerandel's sign," is that the slightest pressure on the body may give rise to severe pain; a hypodermic needle may feel like a red-hot poker, and an accidental blow can cause excruciating discomfort. Some patients present with the symptoms and signs of increased intracranial pressure, convulsions, chorea, athetosis, or Parkinsonism due to basal ganglia involvement. Eventually the victim of sleeping sickness becomes unable to walk, speak, or feed himself; and increasingly cachetic; and dies in coma or from an intercurrent infection.

Some individuals with African trypanosomiasis may remain asymptomatic for long periods even though trypanosomes can be demonstrated in their blood.

Diagnosis

Inexperienced physicians meeting this disease for the first time can make terrible mistakes. Trypanosomal chancres have been treated as bacterial pyogenic lesions; patients with fever, cervical lymphadenopathy, and splenomegaly have been treated for lymphoma, while the encephalitis of sleeping sickness has often gone unrecognized with fatal results. So varied are the manifestations of African trypanosomiasis that any psychiatric or neurological abnormality occurring in a sleeping sickness zone should be considered as due to that disease until proved otherwise. Trypanosomes can be recovered by aspiration from the chancre or from the glands draining the chancre if these are enlarged. Early diagnosis can thus be made before the blood is positive. In Rhodesian disease, parasites are usually readily detectable in the peripheral blood, and the diagnosis can be made by thick film examination. However, *T. gambiense* is less easily found. Greater sensitivity is obtained by microhematocrit centrifugation and by passing larger volumes of blood through anion exchange columns followed by centrifugation of the eluate; field kits for these procedures are available. In Gambiense infection, trypanosomes may be found by lymph node aspiration. In Rhodesiense infection, one can increase the detection rate by rodent inoculation.

After trypanosomes have been identified, lumbar puncture is mandatory, and a white cell count of over 5 per mm^3 and/or a raised protein concentration greater than 25 mg per 100 ml is taken as confirmatory of central nervous system (CNS) involvement.

Double centrifugation techniques will often reveal trypanosomes in the cerebrospinal fluid even when the cell count and protein concentration are normal.

Other helpful, but nonspecific, indicators of possible trypanosome infection include a raised mononuclear cell count in the blood and a raised IgM concentration in either serum or cerebrospinal fluid. For epidemiological surveys, the Card agglutination trypanosomiasis test (CATT) and the Card Indirect agglutination antigen test (CIAT) are available. An antigen-trapping ELISA technique for antigen detection has been developed.

Treatment

Specific chemotherapy is almost 100% effective in African trypanosomiasis if administered in adequate dose early in the disease before involvement of the CNS has occurred. The drug of choice is suramin (Antrypol), which must be given intravenously. A small dose (0.2 g) should be initially administered to test hypersensitivity; if there is no adverse reaction, this is followed by 20 mg per kg bw by slow intravenous (IV) injection on days 1, 3, 7, 14, and 21. Many relatively mild side effects may occur, but the most serious is a nephropathy. The urine must be tested for any significant increase in proteinuria, casts, or red cells before each dose is administered. An alternative drug, for *T. gambiense* infection only, is pentamidine isethionate in a dose of 4 mg per kg bw daily by IV or intramuscular (IM) injection for 10 days.

Until very recently, the only effective treatment for advanced African trypanosomiasis with CNS involvement was melarsoprol, a trivalent arsenical linked to dimercaprol. Unfortunately, this is an extremely toxic drug carrying a mortality in its own right of 1% to 5%. Before therapy, the patient must be first medically rehabilitated as much as possible by correcting dehydration, anemia, and any associated infection. It is a standard practice to also give 3 preliminary doses of suramin to eliminate parasites from the blood.

Melarsoprol, dispensed in 5 ml ampules, each containing 180 mg, is administered by very slow IV injection through a narrow-gauge needle in 3 courses of 3 days, each course separated by 1 week. The doses are 2.5 ml, 3.0 ml, 3.5 ml; then 3.5 ml, 4.0 ml, and 4.5 ml; followed by 5.0 ml, 5.0 ml, and 5.0 ml. The most dangerous side effects are a reactive or a hemorrhagic encephalitis; steroids may be used in an attempt to prevent this reaction. Approximately 80% of patients respond to melarsoprol, but 15% to 20% of these will relapse so that follow-up lumbar punctures are required for up to 2 years following a course of treatment.

Melarsoprol is, obviously, far from being an ideal medication. Alpha-difluoromethylornithine (DFMO; eflornithine) is an important

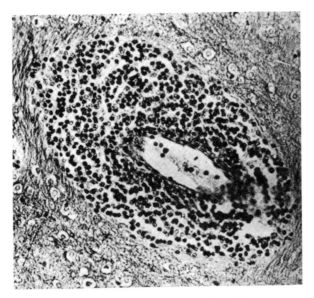

FIGURE 5: Perivascular cuffing in the brain of an African
sleeping sickness victim.

advance, especially for late stage *T. b. gambiense*, which has become
resistant to melarsoprol. The dose is 400 mg per kg in 4 divided doses
at 6 hourly intervals intravenously for 14 days. It is not recommended
for *T. b. rhodesiense* infections. Side effects are reversible and include
diarrhea, anemia, thrombocytopenia, and hair loss. Nifurtimox has
been used in late stage disease in cases where melarsoprol or eflornithine were ineffective.

A new concise treatment schedule with melarsoprol for later-stage
disease reduces the time spent in hospital and the cost of treatment.
The cure rate, mortality, and side effects are similar to the longer classical courses. The dose is 2.2 mg per kg bw melarsoprol daily for 10 days;
prednisolone 1 mg per kg for days 1–7; 0.75 mg on day 8; 0.5 mg on
day 9; and 0.25 mg per kg on day 10. Prednisolone is given to reduce
the risk of arsenical encephalopathy.

Prevention

By the 1950s, Gambiense trypanosomiasis had been largely controlled
by clearing vegetation sheltering tsetse flies along the sides of rivers

and streams, especially at places where man-fly contact was made. Mechanical clearing was supplemented by spraying and by seeking out and treating infected persons. More recently, visually attractive traps, with or without insecticide impregnation and insecticide-impregnated screens, have proved popular and effective.

It should be remembered that many of the great game parks are areas that were originally abandoned because of the unacceptable level of trypanosomiasis among the local population. Tsetse flies hunt by night, feed by day, and are much attracted by moving vehicles. Therefore, those on safari in many parts of East Africa are prime targets, and no effective prophylactic measures are available for visitors to these areas.

American Trypanosomiasis

In 1907, a young Brazilian doctor, Carlos Chagas, aged 28 years, from the Oswaldo Cruz Institute in Rio de Janeiro, was sent to investigate an outbreak of malaria that forced work to be halted on the construction of a new railroad in the Valley of Rio Das Velhas. There, he was shown an insect known as the Barbeiro, a bug that was abundant in all the local houses. In both the feces of this bug and in its hindgut, he found numerous flagellates that he recognized as trypanosomes.

These trypanosomes were unique in having an outsize blephoroplast (kinetoplast), and he named them *Trypanosoma cruzi* in honor of his chief, "a master of unforgettable memory." Returning later to the same area, he found the same parasite in the blood of a cat, and two weeks later, a child from the same house fell ill with a high fever, enlargement of lymph nodes, hepatosplenomegaly, and a most noticeable generalized infiltration of the face. Examination of her blood revealed the same trypanosomes. The girl recovered to outlive Chagas by 32 years.

In every nation of South America and Central America and as far north as Maryland in the United States, *Trypanosoma cruzi* exists as a zoonotic parasite. Where climatic conditions are suitable and man lives in close proximity with appropriate animal reservoirs and insect vectors, Chagas' disease (human American trypanosomiasis) is common. It is conservatively estimated that more than 15 million persons are affected; the majority of cases thus far reported are from Brazil,

Venezuela, and Argentina, and mainly from the poor, rural populations who live in thatched-roof or mud-walled hovels infected with *Triatoma* bugs.

The Parasite

Trypanosoma cruzi resembles the somewhat larger African species of trypanosomes, but differs in the size of the kinetoplast, which may be so large as to distort the cell membrane and produce the "C" configuration that the parasite assumes when dead. Enzyme electrophoresis analysis and kinetoplast DNA profiles have proved useful for the characterization and grouping of zymodemes strains (Z1, Z2, and Z3). These strains have different geographical distributions, transmission cycles, and cause a varying pathology. Z1 is a sylvatic strain causing a natural infection of opossums and other arboreal animals; Z2 is associated with purely domestic transmission by *Triatoma infestans*; Z3, an infection of terrestrial animals, including the nine-banded armadillo, rarely infects man. These parasites are known as stercorian trypanosomes. When ingested by the bug vector, they revert to the epimastigote form in the stomach where they multiply, and then passing down the gut, change into the infective metacyclic form, and are passed to the exterior in the bug feces.

The Vector

The reduvid bug (cone-nosed bug, assassin bug) is an elongated insect, 1 to 3 cm in length of a dull color. The insect's proboscis, when not being used for feeding, is carried under the head and thorax with its tip resting in a groove between the first pair of legs. Both sexes feed rapaciously on animal or human blood, their only source of food. The female lays pink, smooth-shelled, oval, operculated eggs visible with a hand lens. The eggs hatch after 10 days and delicate, light colored, wingless nymphs emerge, which pass through five stages of development and, before each metamorphosis, must obtain a blood meal. Copulation occurs soon after the emergence of the last nymphal instar, and the female starts laying 10 to 14 days after a subsequent blood meal. They feed at night attacking any exposed surface, but the bites are usually painless. A blood feed takes 10 to 20 minutes, and during this time, the bug passes feces infected with trypanosomes on to the skin.

The human becomes infected when rubbing the feces, containing trypanosomes, into the skin. Important vectors include *Triatoma infestans*, *T. braziliense*, *T. dimidiata*, *T. sordida*, *Panstronsylus megistus*, and *Rhodnius prolixus*.

Pathology

Although trypanosomes can enter the skin through the wound made by the biting bug, they may also penetrate the conjunctiva. The infective metacyclic trypanosomes enter tissue histiocytes where they revert to the amastigote form, dividing actively over 5 days before the cells rupture. The released trypomastigotes enter lymphatics, and are carried to lymph nodes and into the blood stream. Tissues involved include those of the reticuloendothelial system; muscle, particularly cardiac fibers; and the neuronal cells of the hollow viscera.

The presence of multiplying amastigotes is accompanied by little cellular reaction. However, following rupture of the cells and liberation of the parasites, the classic histologic picture of acute Chagas' disease develops. Lymphocytes, macrophages, and plasma cells congregate in the tissue around former amastigote nests.

In the chronic stage, detectable parasitemia is unusual, and amastigotes are rarely seen in affected tissues. In the heart, there is a varying degree of loss of ventricular muscle, fibrosis, involvement of the conducting system, dilatation, and the formation of apical aneurysms that rarely burst. In the intestinal tract, destruction of Meissner's and Auerbach's plexuses, and degeneration of the intramural autonomic ganglia, can produce dilatation as well as achalasia of the esophagus and megacolon.

Clinical Features

Infection is usually acquired from the reduvid bug, but may also be transmitted congenitally, by blood transfusion, and by needle-stick accidents in the laboratory. The acute stage is seen mainly in children, and the earliest evidence of infection may be a small, slightly painful, reddish indurated area—a "chagoma"—at the site of the bite. This lesion may persist for months. A painless, nonpitting unilateral facial edema, especially pronounced about the eye, with associated conjunctivitis (Romaña's sign) is considered pathognomonic of Chagas' disease in endemic areas. The local lymph nodes may be enlarged.

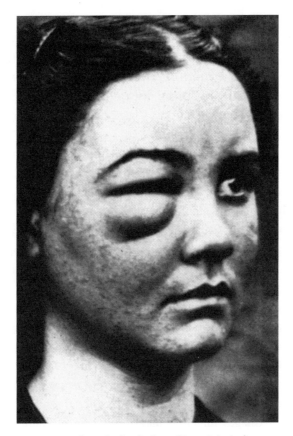

FIGURE 6: Unilateral orbital edema (Romaña's sign), a common initial lesion in Chagas' disease.

After an incubation period of 1 to 2 weeks, systemic manifestations appear. Fever, which may reach hyperpyrexic levels in infants, begins abruptly and may persist for several months, occasionally with a double daily spike. Tachycardia is marked and extends through apyrexial periods. Often, there is an enlargement of lymph nodes and hepatosplenomegaly. In severe infections, there may be acute myocarditis with arrhythmias, pericarditis, or congestive heart failure (CHF), which may prove fatal. Acute meningoencephalitis, trypanosomal orchitis, and thyroiditis are other complications.

Although there is a mortality of 5% to 10%, the acute illness subsides, in a majority of patients, spontaneously after 4 to 8 weeks. Chronic Chagas' disease does not become manifest until many years later, often in early adult life. During the long latent period, infected individuals usually appear to be in normal health; parasitemia is rarely demonstrated, even by xenodiagnosis, although serological tests will be positive. It has become clear that asymptomatic infections with *T. cruzi* can later develop chronic Chagas' disease. By the time patients present with the classic findings of chronic Chagas' disease, they rarely remember the acute phase of the illness.

Chronic Chagas' disease manifests as either a cardiomyopathy, one of the megasyndromes of the intestine, or involvement of both heart and gut. The cardiomyopathy may be mild, manifested only by electrocardiographic abnormalities, such as right bundle branch block, left anterior hemiblock, premature ventricular contractions (PVCs), and T wave changes. More severe manifestations include complete heart block with Stokes-Adams attacks, cardiac arrest, and sudden death. A "sick sinus syndrome" with bradycardia, low cardiac output, and arterial hypotension has been reported, and these patients usually die from biventricular CHF failure and auricular fibrillation. After the more severe manifestations develop, patients usually die within 5 to 6 years. Megaesophagus may be complicated by pulmonary aspiration or esophageal carcinoma. Megacolon is associated with acute sigmoid volvulus, *E. coli* septicemia, and invasive strongyloidiasis.

Congenital Chagas infection may result in a macerated fetus or a jaundiced, edematous, anemic infant with hepatosplenomegaly. Other infected infants appear normal at birth, but later develop tremor, convulsions, spastic paralysis, mental deficiency, and other signs of meningoencephalitis. Chronic megaesophagus has been reported as early as the first year of life. Fever following a blood transfusion in endemic regions should be considered as possibly due to trypanosomiasis.

Diagnosis

Anemia and a peripheral lymphocytosis are common in acute Chagas' disease. Trypanosomes can usually be found without difficulty at this stage. In the latent and chronic phases, parasites are more difficult to demonstrate, and enhancing techniques are required. Xenodiagnosis is a method for detecting a sparse parasitemia. Trypanosome-free reduvid bugs are allowed to feed on the suspected patient, and at intervals

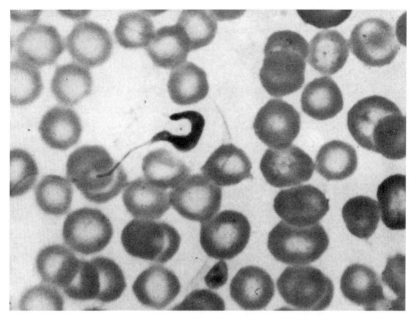

FIGURE 7: Trypanosoma cruzi in typical "C" or "U" configuration in the blood of a patient with acute Chagas' disease.

during the next 2 to 8 weeks, the feces and the guts of the insects are examined for the parasites. A rather less-unpleasant modification is to take 5 ml of heparinized patient's blood and inject it into a membranous bag, which is then placed in a small pot containing the bugs. After feeding, the insects are examined as noted herein. Antibodies to *T. cruzi* may be demonstrated by complement fixation, indirect hemagglutination, indirect fluorescent antibody, tests and by ELISA.

Treatment

Treatment of both acute and chronic Chagas' disease remains unsatisfactory. Nifurtimox (Lampit) 8 to 10 mg per kg bw in 3 divided doses after meals daily for 60 days, or benznidazole 5 mg per kg bw daily for 60 days, has cured some acute cases, but severe side effects are common, especially toward the end of the prolonged drug course, and at least 20% of parasites remain resistant. The addition of allopurinol in a dose of 7 to 10 mg per kg bw may increase therapeutic efficacy.

Current chemotherapy in chronic Chagas' disease is unsatisfactory, and most treatment is only symptomatic. Standard therapy for arrhythmias and CHF with cardiac drugs may be temporarily helpful and pacemakers as well as cardiac defibrillators (ACIDs) to prevent sudden death may assist those Chagas patients with heart block. Cholinergic drugs and rectosigmoidectomy are of use in managing those with megacolon, while mechanical dilatation and surgery can be helpful in those with esophageal achalasia or distention.

Epidemiology and Prevention

Chagas' disease is primarily an infection of subsistence farmers and their families living in remote homesteads in rural areas. The local adobe houses with thatch roofs provide ideal conditions for the triatomid vector bugs. Preventive measures include regular, repeated residual insecticide spraying of houses and outhouses. Until the bugs are eradicated, people should sleep under mosquito nets. A more permanent measure, probably cheaper in the long run, is the replacement of these primitive dwellings with stone houses, plastered walls, and metal or tiled roofs. All blood donors from endemic areas should be screened by serological tests, and blood from these donors should be stored for 10 days before use. In the United States, an estimated 25,000 to 100,000 persons and 1 in 25,000 blood donors may be infected with *T. cruzi*. In South America, Central America, and Mexico, 16 to 18 million people are infected; and the disease accounts for, on average, 50,000 deaths annually. High migration levels of people from Latin America to other parts of the world have turned Chagas' disease into a global problem in recent years. The elimination of Chagas' disease is a WHO global goal, and the disease has already been eradicated in some countries in South America.

Leishmaniases

The leishmaniases are hemoflagellate protozoal infections of animals and man, which in the Old World, are endemic in a broad belt of arid lands stretching through the Mediterranean, northeast Africa, the Middle East, southern Russia, Pakistan, India, and China. In the New

World, they are endemic in the forest regions of Central America and South America.

The Parasite

In the vertebrate host, the parasite occurs in the amastigote form, an inert-looking round or oval body about the size of a blood platelet. On staining with Giemsa, the cytoplasm appears blue, and there are two deeply red/purple staining chromatin bodies: the larger being the nucleus; and the smaller rod-shaped body, the kinetoplast. In the sand-fly vectors and on culture, the parasites take up the promastigote form.

Leishmania causing disease in humans occur as many different strains, each differing in its reservoir, vector, and geographic location; and in the pathological lesions to which it gives rise. Although all strains are similar in morphological appearance, some may be differentiated by their behavior on culture, their position in the sandfly, and by the lesions that they produce in laboratory animals. More precise differentiation can now be obtained by isoenzyme electrophoresis, by reactivity with monoclonal antibodies, and by hybridization of kinetoplast DNA. This differention can have considerable clinical, therapeutic, and epidemiological importance. At least four leishmanial species have been identified as etiologic agents of visceral disease (kala azar), and more than one-dozen strains are associated with cutaneous and mucocutaneous lesions in man.

The Vector

Sandflies—*Phlebotomus*, *Lutomyia*, and *Psychodopygus*—are small, delicately proportioned flies 2 to 3 mm in length. They are light yellow or gray in color with large conspicuous eyes. The legs are long and slender, giving the insect an appearance of walking on stilts. They have very poor powers of flight, tend to be confined to areas immediately around their breeding sites, and are very sensitive to the effects of residual insecticides. The female requires animal or human blood for the maturing of each batch of eggs. Amastigotes ingested in these blood feeds convert to the promastigote form in the gut of the sandfly, and this is followed by rapid multiplication. After about two weeks, small unattached, nondividing forms reach the mouth parts of the sandfly and are injected into vertebrate hosts in a subsequent blood feed.

Pathology

When promastigotes are injected into man, they are rapidly taken up by macrophages in which they revert to the amastigote form. What then happens depends upon the strain of the parasite and on the cell-mediated immune response of the host. Probably in most instances, the parasites are destroyed or at least contained, the only evidence of infection having taken place being a positive leishmanin skin test. In other instances, the parasite multiplies locally within the macrophages to cause a cutaneous lesion; other strains, although they may also cause an initial insignificant local lesion, disseminate in the reticuloendothelial cells of the body to cause visceral leishmaniasis. Yet other strains may cause late lesions affecting the nasoooropharynx.

Diagnosis

Confirmation of the diagnosis of leishmaniases is best given by demonstration of the parasite following aspiration of fluid from infected tissue. Aspirates may also be cultured, the original NNN medium now being superceded by various modifications of Schneider's Drosophila insect medium in which promastigotes develop and multiply within 2 to 3 days. Parasites may also be demonstrated following hamster inoculation. The leishmanin test, a dermal sensitivity test analogous to the tuberculin test, will also provide support for a diagnosis in certain circumstances. The characteristic histopathologic features are best seen on biopsy sections stained with H & E; amastigote forms must be identified in the section for confirmation.

Treatment

Certain mild forms of cutaneous leishmaniasis require no specific treatment, but most forms of leishmaniasis will respond to treatment with pentavalent antimony when given in adequate dosage. This is given as sodium stibogluconate (Pentostam) or meglumine antimoniate (Glucantime) in a dose of 20 mg per kg bw daily by IV or IM injection for 20 to 30 days.

Visceral Leishmaniasis

In the early part of the nineteenth century, a fatal fever was reported from the Central District of Bengal. People developed a relapsing hyperpyrexia associated with generalized wasting, massive splenomegaly, and hyperpigmentation of the skin. Epidemics seemed to occur in 10-year cycles. In 1900, a soldier was invalided back to England with this fever, and at autopsy, Major William Leishman found enormous numbers of round or oval bodies, 2 to 3 micrometers in diameter, in splenic smears. When in 1903, a report of this finding reached Captain Charles Donovan in Madras, he described how he had found similar bodies in smears taken from the enlarged spleens of Indian patients who had been thought to have died of malaria. He also related how "yesterday I had occasion to puncture *in vitam* the spleen of an Indian boy aged 12 years suffering from an irregular pyrexia, but with no malarial parasites in his peripheral blood, and found identical bodies in the blood of the spleen." It was Ronald Ross who named the new protozoa "the Leishman-Donovan body." Another pioneer in tropical medicine, Charles Nicolle, working in Tunisia in the early part of the 20th century, suggested the zoonotic nature of epidemics with the domestic dog as the local reservoir. Of the 500,000 estimated new cases per year, one-half are thought to occur in India.

Pathology

Visceral leishmaniasis is characterized by the dissemination of amastigotes throughout the reticuloendothelial system of the body, particularly in the spleen, bone marrow, lymph nodes, liver, and small intestine. The diffuse nature of the disease appears to be associated with the host's deficient cell-mediated immune response to the parasite; the leishmanin test is always negative; and, in endemic regions, kala azar is not an uncommon opportunistic infection in patients with AIDS. Most of the cases seen in Europe are now in patients with AIDS.

An ineffective humoral immune response is reflected in the production of excessive amounts of polyclonal, nonspecific, nonprotective IgG immunoglobulins, and the serum albumin concentration falls. Leucopenia and thrombocytopenia are characteristic, and a normochromic, normocytic anemia follows.

Clinical Features

Infection is usually transmitted by the bite of a sandfly, but it may also follow blood transfusion. The incubation period varies from 10 days to several years, but is commonly 3 to 6 months. A common presentation in expatriates is a sudden onset of chills and a high swinging fever accompanied by drenching sweats. In about 20% of these patients, the temperature chart reveals a double rise every 24 hours. In spite of the high fever, patients feel reasonably well and can often see no reason why they should be confined to bed. There may be increased skin pigmentation, and the spleen is enlarged and firm.

In the indigenous inhabitants of endemic areas, the clinical presentation is more varied. The onset may be insidious with a low-grade fever that may later become irregular, remittent, intermittent, or continuous. Patients, especially children, complain of pain in the left hypochondrium and increasing abdominal distension, both from an enlarged spleen. Cough may be a prominent symptom and may or may not be associated with pulmonary tuberculosis. The skin may be hyperpigmented and rough; the hair sparse and brittle; and there may be edema of the legs, with purpura. Jaundice may also be present. Kirk, in Sudan, described two classic polar types of visceral leishmaniasis: patients who presented with acute onset of high fever and severe constitutional symptoms, but with little or no obvious splenic enlargement, responded rapidly to treatment, but died early if untreated. Other patients presented with chronic ill health, but only occasional attacks of fever, had very large spleens, responded poorly to treatment, and usually died of intercurrent infection. Asymptomatic and subclinical infections are common.

Leishmania and HIV–coinfection persons present in an atypical way: Splenomegaly may be absent; cutaneous and mucocutaneous lesions are common; and nodular or ulcerative lesions may occur in the tongue, larynx, esophagus, stomach, rectum, and lungs. Response to treatment is poor; 30% of patients die within 1 month of treatment.

Diagnosis

There is usually a well-marked leukopenia and thrombocytopenia, and the erythrocyte sedimentation rate (ESR) is very high. The serum albumin is reduced and the globulins much elevated, the rise being in the IgG gamma globulin fraction. The most satisfactory method of confirming the diagnosis is by demonstration of amastigotes in a splenic aspirate. To attempt a percutaneous puncture, the spleen must be palpable at least 3 cm below the costal margin, the prothrombin time not more than 5.5 longer than the control, and the platelet count should exceed 40,000/mm^3. A 21-gauge needle is attached to a 5 ml glass syringe, and both must be sterile and completely dry. The needle is made to penetrate the skin midway between the edges of the spleen and 2 to 4 cm below the costal margin. It is then aimed upward at an angle of 45° to the abdominal wall. The patient holds his breath, and the needle is then plunged into the spleen and immediately withdrawn with a quick in-and-out movement, suction being maintained throughout. A few drops of aspirate are obtained, some of which is immediately inoculated into Schneider's medium and the rest smeared onto clean glass slides, fixed with methanol, and stained with Giemsa.

Alternative, less satisfactory, but often preferred, sources for aspiration are the bone marrow and lymph nodes. Various serological tests are available: direct and indirect agglutination, immunofluorescence, or ELISA. New techniques include monoclonal antibodies nucleic acid hybridization and polymerase chain reaction (PCR). In all forms of kala azar, the leishmanin skin test (Montenegro test), which measures delayed hypersensitivity, is negative but will become positive some months after cure.

The K39 test, which is commercially available, was shown to be 100% sensitive and 98% specific in India; however, in Sudan and Nepal, its specificity was poor. A nested PCR assay and PCR-ELISA of blood are available and avoid the need for bone marrow or splenic aspiration. A direct agglutination test (DAT) using urine samples has been developed and compares favorably with that of urine ELISA.

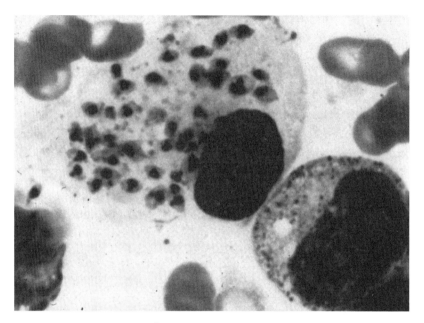

FIGURE 8: Bone marrow smear from a patient with visceral leishmaniasis. Numerous L-D bodies are found within momcytic cells.

Treatment

Standard treatment is with Pentostam or Glucantime in a dose of 20 mg antimony per kg for 20 to 42 days by IV or IM injection. If effective, the fever will fall within 7 days, and the spleen begin to regress after 2 weeks. Clinical improvement should be obvious, and a reappearance of eosinophils is a good sign. However, relapse may occur, particularly in patients who have received suboptimal treatment; in these patients, the parasite may have become relatively resistant. In the state of Bihar, 37% 64% of newly diagnosed visceral leishmaniasis cases fail to respond or relapse after conventional pentavalent therapy. Relapses should be treated with the same dose of Pentostam given for 60 days, and such cases are being increasingly reported from India. A new compound, miltefosine, has been approved for therapy in several countries but is not yet available, for example, in the United States.

In cases of visceral leishmaniasis unresponsive to antimony—and such cases are being increasing reported from India—pentamidine can be used. A dose of 4 mg per kg twice weekly IM is given until parasitological cure is obtained. In India, it has been combined with a course of antimony, but side effects were considerable although a high cure rate was obtained.

Three lipid formulations of amphotericin B are available: liposomal amphotericin B (Ambisome), amphotericin B cholesterol dispersion (Amphocil), and amphotericin B lipid complex (Abelcet R). Treatment courses are short; the drugs are safe and very effective but expensive. The dose is 3 mg per kg daily on days 1 to 5, day 14, and 21.

Aminosidine (paromomycin) in a dose of 12 to 15 mg per kg once daily for 17 to 20 days in combination with antimony proved effective and safe in southern Sudan and India.

Miltefosine is a highly effective oral treatment for visceral leishmaniasis. In India, 100 mg per day (2.5 mg per kg per day in children) for 4 weeks achieved cure rates of 95%. It is cheap. Unfortunately, it is abortifacient and teratogenetic, and may reduce male fertility. It also has a long half-life. Its use is excluded in women of childbearing age.

Hyperalimentation to correct malnutrition, blood transfusion for severe anemia, the maintenance of satisfactory oral hygiene, and the concurrent therapy of any associated infection or infections are other very important elements in the overall treatment of patients with kala azar.

Epidemiology

Several species of *L. donovani* cause kala azar in different parts of the world. The illness is very similar, but the epidemiology differs.

Table 3 shows the epidemiology of kala azar.

Table 3.   Epidemiology of kala azar

Parasite	Location	Vector	Reservoir
L. d. donovani	India	*P. argentipes*	Man
L. d. donovani	Sudan	*P. orientalis*	Ground rodent
L. d. infantum	Mediterranean	*P. perniciosus*	Dogs, foxes
L. d. chagasi	Latin America	*Lu. longipalpis*	Dogs, foxes

In India, there appears to be no animal reservoir of infection, and the disease is transmitted by peridomestic sandflies from human to human. In Sudan, the reservoir of infection are Nile grass rats and other rodents which, during the hot arid days, cohabit in the relatively cool, humid environment of the deep cracks in the black cotton soil with *Phlebotomus orientalis*. In the Mediterranean and in South America, dogs and foxes form the reservoir of infection, and the human victims are mainly infants and young children. In Asia, along the Great Silk Road, kala azar is transmitted from dogs to man as in the Mediterranean, while along the China coast, the epidemiology is similar to that in India.

Measures to protect the population of endemic regions will differ according to the epidemiological situation, but where applicable, residual insecticide spraying can be very effective. It is important that cattle sheds and chicken houses should also be sprayed. Where domestic dog reservoirs exist, they should be treated or destroyed. Personal protection is accomplished by reasonably simple, common sense rules: wearing suitable clothing in the evening because sandflies are unable to penetrate even the most flimsy garments; and by sleeping upstairs, where sandflies cannot reach because of their limited powers of flight. No vaccine or prophylactic chemotherapy is available.

In addition to kala azar, *Leishmania donovani* infection can produce other pathological conditions:

Post Kala Azar Dermal Leishmaniasis. Apparent cure of kala azar may be followed by a cutaneous eruption, which takes the form of either skin nodules or depigmented macules. The lesions contain masses of amastigotes, and affected individuals are important sources for infection of sandflies. In India, where this condition appears to be especially common, lesions usually appear about 2 years after treatment of kala azar, but sometimes no history of infection can be elicited. In Sudan, the onset is usually much more rapid. In both countries, the condition is relatively resistant to therapy, and full doses of antimony may have to be given for prolonged periods.

Oriental Sore. *L. donovani* can cause cutaneous lesions similar to oriental sores. This has been documented in Sudan, particularly among those better protected by adequate nutrition. Now that parasites can be more accurately identified, it has also become clear that *L. infantum* in the Mediterranean is a common cause of skin lesions even in the absence of disseminated disease. Chemoprophylaxes for HIV/AIDS patients has been promoted as an important adjunct in Brazil and in a number of Mediterranean countries.

Oronasal Leishmaniasis. In Sudan, and occasionally in India, *L. donovani* infection may present with mucosal lesions. Two types are seen: a fungating ulcerated granulomatous tumor containing plentiful amastigotes, and a diffuse ulcerative lesion in which parasites may be demonstrated only following culture of biopsy material. Both these lesions respond well to treatment with Pentostam.

Lymphatic Leishmaniasis. *L. donovani* infection may present with only an enlargement of lymph nodes, usually in the cervical region, and without any constitutional upset. The histological appearance of these nodes is very similar to sarcoidosis, but parasites can be demonstrated after a thorough search or following culture.

Cutaneous and Mucocutaneous Leishmaniasis
Old World Cutaneous Leishmaniasis

Leishmania tropica

In 1856, Alexander Russell, the physician to a community of prosperous English merchants in Syria, described a condition known locally as the "Aleppo evil." It affected native children, as well as almost all European adults, within a few months of their arrival in the area. The lesion started as a small, red, painless pimple, commonly disregarded, but slowly increased to a 12 mm diameter circular sore. After some months, it might scurvy on top or, alternatively, enlarge to form a superficial ulcer with a livid border. The lesion remained painless and usually healed in 8 to 12 months, but many beautiful faces were disfigured.

L. tropica is mainly an urban infection. The primary reservoir is man although dogs may also be victims. The main vector is *Phlebotomus papatasi*, the domestic sandfly, which breeds in wall cracks, debris, heaps of rubbish, and privies. They bite man when they emerge at night in search of food. In recent years, the incidence of infection has fallen sharply as a result of the application of residual insecticides.

Pathology. On histological sections, the early lesion consists of a nodule with many macrophages and numerous amastigotes. Later lesions contain an exudative cellular reaction consisting of lymphocytes and plasma cells, which is accompanied by lysis of macrophages, local necrosis, a sharp fall in the number of amastigotes, and local ulceration.

Clinical Features. The incubation period varies from 1 month to several months. What seems at first to be a simple insect bite fails to heal and an itchy papule develops, enlarges peripherally, and becomes covered with fine papery scales. The lesion may develop no further; in other cases, the scales become moist, and the nodule breaks down to

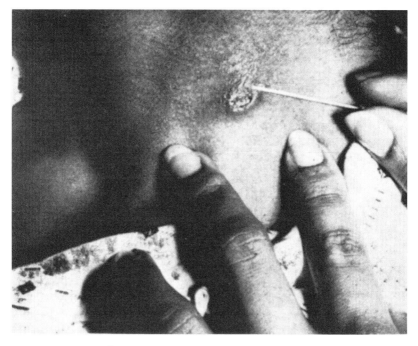

FIGURE 9: Aspirating for amastigotes through healthy skin adjacent to an oriental sore.

form an ulcer that oozes serous fluid. Ulcers are typically shallow and encrusted, with a sharp, elevated, and indurated border surrounded by a narrow zone of erythema. Removal of the crust leaves a bleeding granular surface. Lesions may be single or multiple, but are limited to areas of the skin exposed to sandfly bites; they are never seen on the hairy scalp. Spontaneous healing occurs after 2 to 20 months leaving a pink or depigmented, depressed scar which, on the face, is often disfiguring.

An uncommon manifestation of L. tropica infection is chronic lupoid leishmaniasis, which is a deforming condition clinically resembling lupus vulgaris. A butterfly-shaped flat scar with peripheral nodules develops on the face, and the condition may persist for up to 20 years with periods of activation each summer. Biopsy reveals epitheliod tubercles without lymphatic infiltration. Amastigotes can rarely be demonstrated. The leishmanin skin test is strongly positive. Successful therapy requires larger doses and a longer course of Pentostam.

Diagnosis. The diagnosis of L. tropica infection is usually confirmed by passing a dry, sterile needle through adjacent normal skin into the margin of the lesion and aspirating a few drops of fluid. This material is then stained with Giemsa for microscopic examination, placed on Schneider's or NNN culture media, or injected intraperitoneally into a golden hamster. The biopsy picture is classical; amastigotes should be sought beneath the ulcerated dermis. A positive leishmanin test is a helpful guide, especially in expatriates.

Treatment. Many L. tropica lesions heal without specific chemotherapy. Local care, including debridement and cleaning of the ulcer, and use of antibiotic cream to control secondary bacterial infection, is often adequate. With multiple, large, and especially with facial lesions, a course of intravenous Pentostam is warranted.

Leishmania major

The lesions caused by this parasite are similar to those seen in L. tropica infections, but tend to be more often numerous, florid, and moist, and are accompanied by obvious lymph node enlargement. Nodular and verrucose forms are also described. The ulcers tend to mature more rapidly and heal more quickly, but are associated with more severe scarring. In contrast with L. tropica, this is a rural infection; the reservoir are ground rodents, such as the gerbil. The vectors, P. papatasi and P. duboscqui, shelter from the heat and aridity in rodent burrows, coming out only at night to feed on unfortunate humans.

Leishmania ethiopica

An unusual form of cutaneous leishmaniasis occurs in the highlands of Ethiopia and in the Mount Kenya region, the reservoir being the rock hyrax (rabbits) and the vectors being P. lonqipes and P. pedtfer. The lesions range from simple tropical ulcers to a gross dissemination of nonulcerative nodules or plaques, particularly on the face and limbs. The lesions, which do not remit spontaneously, are very disfiguring. There is a clinical and immunological resemblance to lepromatous leprosy, but biopsy reveals intense infiltration with macrophages teeming with amastigotes. Lymphocytes are absent and the leishmanin test is negative. Pentostam therapy, even in high doses for long periods, has not been satisfactory and alternate drugs, including Lomidine, have proved quite toxic for the duration of treatment required.

New World Cutaneous Leishmaniasis

In Latin America, cutaneous leishmaniasis is endemic from Mexico in the north to Argentina in the south. The first major outbreak occurred when labor forces penetrated into the deep primary forest constructing roads, railroads, and mining camps. Infection is with two species of Leishmania—L. mexicana and L. braziliensis—and it is of clinical importance to distinguish these species.

The Parasite

L. mexicana amastigotes and promastigotes are large and relatively easy to culture in simple blood agar media; and, in the sandfly, the promastigotes are confined to the midgut and foregut (suprapylorian). When inoculated into the skin of laboratory hamsters or mice, they produce

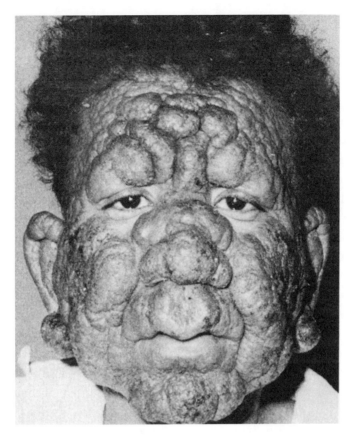

FIGURE 10: An Egyptian with diffuse cutaneous leishmaniasis simulating leprosy.

large histiocytoma-like lesions containing abundant amastigotes. On the other hand, *L. braziliensis* parasites are smaller and difficult to maintain in culture; and, in the sandfly, initially establish themselves in the hindgut as round or pear-shaped promastigotes (peripylorian). The parasites later migrate forward to the midgut where multiplication takes place. When inoculated into the hamster skin, this species produces slow growing, inconspicuous nodules that contain scanty amastigotes.

Each strain contains several subspecies differing in their animal reservoir, sandfly vector, and the lesion produced in man. These subspecies may be differentiated by enzyme electrophoresis and study of the kinetoplast DNA.

Table 4 presents the epidemiology of American leishmaniasis.

Clinical Features

In general, *L. mexicana* infections are manifest by cutaneous lesions very similar to those seen in Old World cutaneous leishmaniasis.

L. m. mexicana is the cause of the "Chiclero ulcer," which is a destructive granulomatous lesion affecting the ears of men who collect latex from sapodilla trees in the jungles of Latin America for the manufacture of chewing gum. *L. m. amazonensis* and *L. m. perfanoi* infections can produce a diffuse cutaneous leishmaniasis similar to that seen in Ethiopia. Similarly, *L. b. braziliensis* infections are usually associated with cutaneous ulceration, often with rather prominent lymphatic involvement, but can occasionally cause far more extensive lesions. *Leishmania b. braziliensis* is the most important parasite causing American cutaneous leishmaniasis, not only because it is the most widespread and common strain, but because a late manifestation is nasooropharyngeal ulceration (espundia) that, untreated, results in a mutilating facial deformity, severe social consequences, and, not uncommonly, death. It is endemic from Panama in the north to Argentina in the south. The vector is *Psychodopygus wellcomei*, an aggressive sandfly that

Table 4. Epidemiology of American leishmaniasis

Parasite	Reservoir	Vector
Leishmania mexicana		
L. m. mexicana	Tree rodents	*Lu olmeca*
L. m. amazonensis	Ground rodents	*Lu flaviscutella*
L. m. pifanoi	Unknown	Unknown
L. m. venezualensis	Unknown	Unknown
Leishmania braziliensis		
L. b. braziliensis	Unknown	*Psy. wellcomei*
L. b. guyanensis	Sloths, anteaters	*Lu umbritalis*
L. b. panamensis	Marmosets/spiny rats	*Lu trapidoi*
L. b. peruviana	Dogs	*Lu verrucarim*

attacks man viciously at night and during the day in overcast conditions. The reservoir of infection remains unknown.

The incubation period may be as short as 15 days. The lesions, which occur most often on the lower anterior tibial third of the leg, are characterized by early necrosis, resulting in craterform extensive ulcers that are slow to heal. Less commonly, the lesions appear as warty verrucose excrescences or plaques. In about one-third of cases, the lesions are multiple.

In approximately 2% 5% of patients, the acute cutaneous lesions are followed after an interval of 2 to 20 years by granulomatous involvement of the nose, mouth, pharynx, and larynx, usually starting as a crusting on the anterior nasal septum. Patients may complain of nasal blockage, epistaxis, excessive secretion, or even the passage of pieces of tissue, while others present with pain in the nose, deformity, or inflammation. Granulomatous plaques, ulcers, or polyps may be seen on the septal epithelium, and partial or complete loss of the cartilaginous septum may follow with perforation. Cartilaginous collapse may

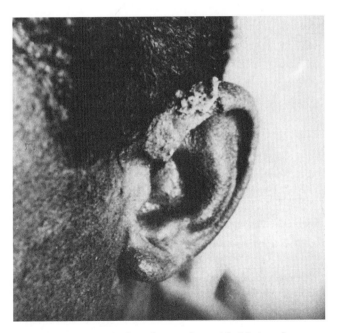

FIGURE 11: An acute Chiclero ulcer on the ear of a Mexican farmer.

result in broadening and flattening to produce the so-called "tapir nose."

Granulomata may also appear on the palate as rather hard protuberances that later become eroded, and the process may spread backward to the soft palate, uvula, and pharynx; or, less commonly, forward to involve the gums and upper lip. Laryngeal involvement may be manifest by a hoarse voice and a brassy cough. The condition is painless, and the course unpredictable, but it may end in gross destruction of tissue and severe mutilation. The diagnosis depends on the clinical features and the demonstration, if possible, of the parasite. The leishmanin test will be positive, and except in severely malnourished patients, antibodies are demonstrated in the serum. Even if no amastigotes are found, the histology of a biopsy may be helpful.

Treatment

In endemic areas of South America and Central America, it is, therefore, obvious that because of the unpredictable and latent dangers of espundia, even minor primary ulcers should, whenever possible, be treated with a full course of Pentostam or Glucantime. Patients should then be followed up to ensure that the antibody titer is falling. Late lesions will also respond to courses of antimonials that must be maintained until there is no longer evidence of activity. Very few patients now require treatment with amphotericin B. Reconstructive facial surgery is often necessary if patients are to return to community life.

Amebiasis

Entamoeba histolytica is a protozoal parasite of man and a wide range of nonhuman primates. The organism was first described in St. Petersburg by Losch in 1875; in 1903, it was distinguished by Schaudinn from the more common, nonpathogenic organism *Entamoeba coli*. Human infection has been reported in all countries but is much more frequent in the tropics and subtropics. It is estimated that as many as 500 million new infections occur every year; in many cases, the parasite appears to live in the human intestine as a harmless commensal. When the organism is invasive, however, victims suffer greatly, and physicians often compound the situation by errors in both diagnosis and therapy. In recent years, alterations in host resistance have even further complicated the clinical challenge of amebiasis. In those patients in whose resistance is altered by steroids, oncologic chemotherapy, or HIV/AIDS, amebic infection can develop in a fulminant, even fatal, fashion.

The Parasite

The trophozoite forms of *E. histolytica*, 15 to 30 microns in size, have clear ectoplasmic borders, characteristic nuclei with minute central karysomes, and uniformly stained rings of peripheral chromatin of even thickness. They display motility through protrusion of pseudopodia. Trophozoites live in the lumen of the bowel, mainly cecum and ascending colon, where the contents are liquid. In this anaerobic environment, they feed on bacteria and fecal debris, and multiply by binary fission.

As the parasites pass down the colon to regions where the contents become more solid, they cease to feed and then round up and secrete a tough wall to form cysts 10 to 20 microns across, first with single nuclei and ultimately with four. The nuclei remain unchanged, but the cytoplasm of the cysts develop a glycogen vacuole as well as two refractile rod-shaped structures known as chromodial bars. The cysts passed in the stools are resistant to environmental conditions and can remain viable for weeks.

Infection is acquired by ingestion of cysts. They pass unscathed through the acid contents of the stomach, but in the alkaline medium of the small intestine, the cyst walls weaken, and from each cyst, a four-nucleated metacyst squeezes out. Almost immediately, the cytoplasm divides so that four separate metacysts are produced, each of which divides again before reaching the colon. Trophozoites and cysts may be cultured on special media, such as that of Robinson.

It has now become clear that there are many strains of *Entamoeba histolytica*, only some of which are pathogenic. The pathogenic, invasive strains may be identified after culture by starch gel electrophoresis with the enzymes hexokinase and phosphoglutamase, and by monoclonal antibody studies. Using these techniques, some 22 zymodemes have been identified, but only a minority of these have been associated with tissue invasiveness. Biochemical, immunological, and genetic data has now established that these are two species with similar morphological characteristics: *E. histolytica and E. dispar.* Only *E. histolytica* is capable of causing invasive disease, which is often associated with high levels of specific antibodies. Finding trophozoites with ingested red blood cells suffices as a basis for treatment. Other minor protozoa, whose main significance is that they are often confused by inexperienced technicians with *E. histolytica*, can be found in Figure 12. *Giardia lambia* is discussed with traveler's diarrhea.

Amebic Dysentery

Pathology

Invasive trophozoites enter the colonic mucosal crypts where, by secreting cytolytic enzymes, they cause local necrosis, the cell debris being engulfed by the parasites. Small, discrete, flask-shaped ulcers are produced, which due to the resistance of the muscularis mucosa, usually remain superficial and spare the intervening mucosa. However, in patients with impaired resistance, the lesions become so extensive that the whole colon can be involved and become extremely friable. In such patients, seepage of lumen contents into the peritoneum, frank perforation, and toxic megacolon are dangerous complications.

Clinical Features

The incubation period can rarely be determined exactly, but is usually measured in days rather than hours after exposure, and can be several months and even years. There are two polar types of amebic dysentery with intermediate variations. In well-fed, previously healthy North American and Europeans living under comfortable conditions, the usual presentation is with mild diarrhea, 3 to 4 loose stools being passed daily. These may be streaked with blood and mucus. The diarrhea is often intermittent and may be interspersed with periods of constipation. There may be little or no constitutional upset, fever, pain, or tenesmus, and these individuals usually remain ambulant. On physical examination, some pain may be elicited by deep pressure over the sigmoid or cecal areas.

By contrast, in malnourished people, pregnant women, children after measles, soldiers living under arduous conditions, and immunocompromised patients, a fulminating dysenteric disease may occur. Diarrhea, with 10 to 20 liquid, bloody, foul-smelling stools daily is often accompanied by fever, severe weakness, dehydration, tenesmus, generalized abdominal pain, and vomiting. Peritonitis or toxic megacolon may complicate the picture. The bowel wall is so friable that careless clinical palpation or endoscopic examination may cause it to rupture. The mortality may reach 50%. Between these two clinical extremes, all grades of severity are seen. One presentation, which gives particular difficulty in diagnosis, is almost indistinguishable from ulcerative colitis. The clinician must remember the fecal oral transmission cycle in treating an infected person. The intimacy of sexual life, for example, is often associated with the spread of infection to a partner, and a "ping pong" situation can develop, allowing perpetuation of infection in a household.

PARASITE	TROPHOZOITE	CYST	SYMPTOMS	TREATMENT
DIENTAMEBA FRAGILIS			NONE	NOT INDICATED
ENTAMEBA COLI			NONE	NOT INDICATED
ENDOLIMAX NANA			NONE	NOT INDICATED
IODAMEBA BUTSCHLII			NONE	NOT INDICATED
CHILIMASTRIX MENILI			NONE	NOT INDICATED

			OCCASIONAL DIARRHEA AND CHOLECYSTITS (?) STEATTORHEA	METRONIDAZOLE NITAZOXANIDE
GIARDIA LAMBLIA				
TRICHOMONAS HOMINIS		NOT KNOWN	NONE	NONE
BALANTIDIUM COLI			DIARRHEA DYSETERY	UNSATISFACTORY ARSENICALS ANTIBIOTICS DIIODOQUIN

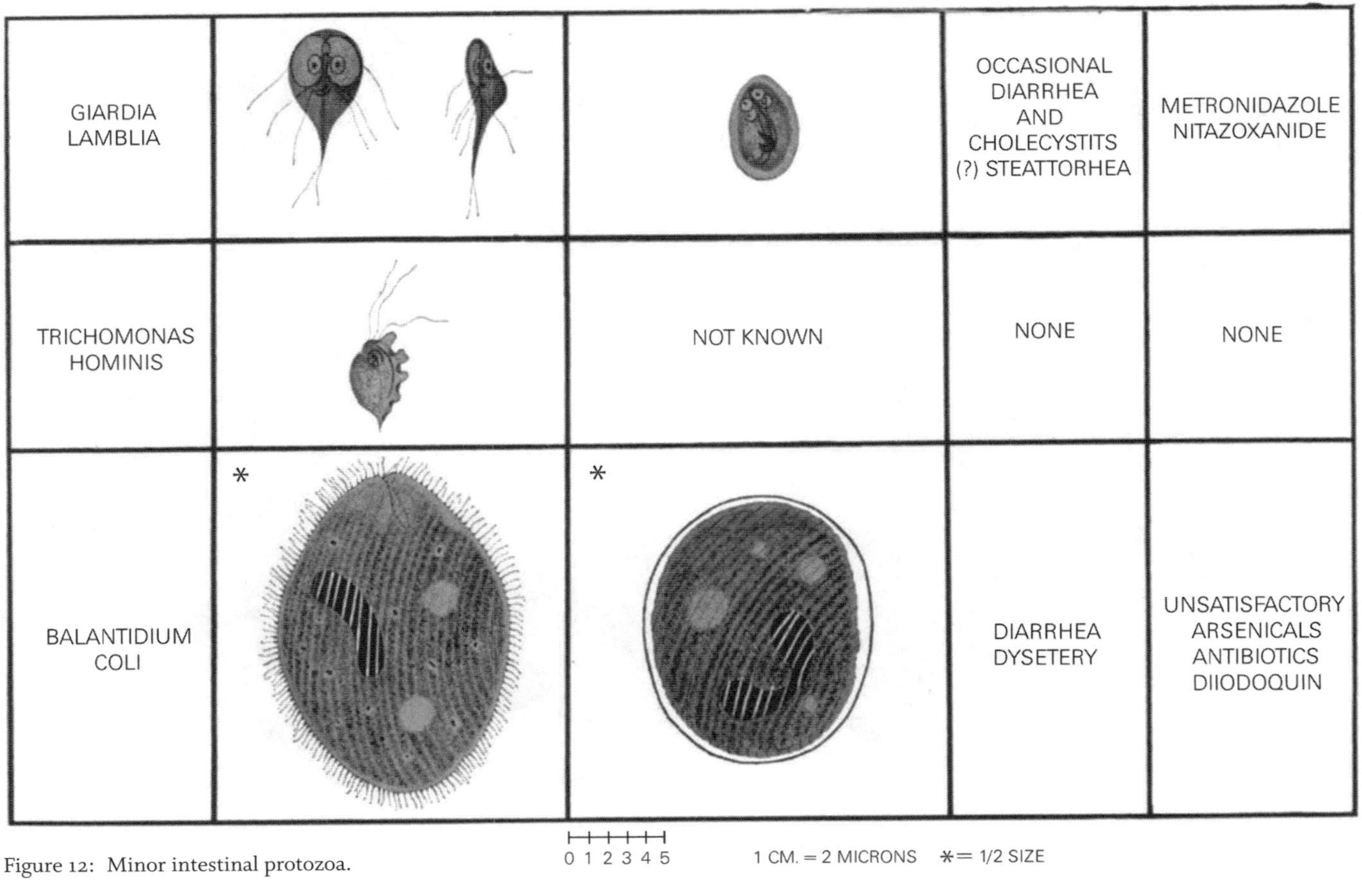

* = 1/2 SIZE   1 CM. = 2 MICRONS

0 1 2 3 4 5

Figure 12: Minor intestinal protozoa.

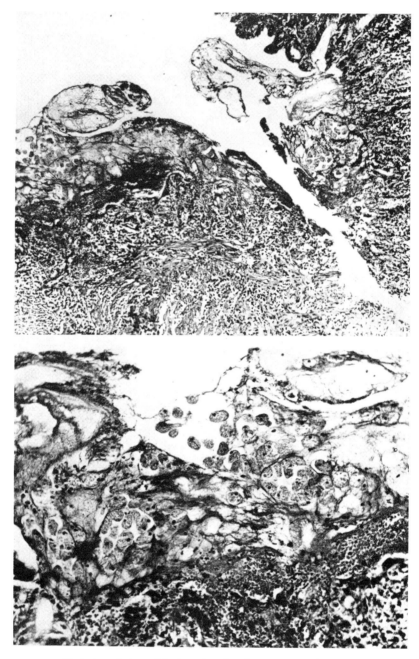

FIGURE 13: Flask-shaped ulcer of the large bowel with extension in the submucosa. Nests of E. histolytica can be seen on the mucosal edge.

Diagnosis

The milder type of amebic dysentery can often best be confirmed in the side room of a clinic or hospital ward. A loopful of blood stained mucus is taken from the surface of the bowel wall via the sigmoidoscope or from freshly passed stool and then emulsified in normal saline on a slide; a coverslip is applied, and the stool is examined with a 10X objective. Motile trophozoites may be recognized, which contain red blood cells "rolling over each other like snooker balls in a bag." These must be differentiated from large macrophages, which may also contain red cells but have large irregular nuclei. An iron hematoxylin stain may be used to preserve smears. Stools sent to the laboratory should be examined immediately or placed in polyvinyl alcohol and merthiolate iodine formalin (MIF) or sodium acetate formalin (SAF). Trophozoites rapidly round up and become immobile. They are, therefore, recognized most readily in fresh material, but an immunofluorescent stain may be helpful in identifying trophozoites in specimens submitted for later analysis.

The clinician must remember that the stool is merely a convenient vehicle passing by. Ameba live in the bowel wall. Direct observation, especially in chronic cases, is preferable to merely examining fecal specimens. Proctoscopy and sigmoidoscopy are essential procedures for the tropicalist, and trophozoites that are difficult to detect in stool studies may be readily obtained from direct scrapings of ulcers. The typical sigmoidoscopic appearance in amebiasis is of small discrete ulcers covered with white or yellow exudate on a background of normal mucosa. Because amebic ulcers can extend laterally in the submucosa (flask-shaped), endoscopic biopsies are usually contraindicated. Casual biopsies can—and do—result in perforation. Many factors adversely affect the chance of detecting amebae, and patients must be questioned regarding these interfering factors (see Table 5) before accepting a "negative" parasitologic result.

The diagnosis of the more severe types of amebic dysentery may, ironically, be most difficult. As noted, sigmoidoscopy can be dangerous, and the appearances of the bowel wall may be indistinguishable from that seen in severe ulcerative colitis. Moreover, patients with ulcerative colitis may also be infected with nonpathogenic *Entamoeba coli* and may

Table 5. Factors that interfere with parasitological examination of feces

Factor	Substance
Antidiarrheal preparations	Bismuth, kaolin
Radiographic procedures	Barium sulfate
Biologically active drugs	Sulphonamides, antibiotic agents, antiprotozoal drugs, anthelminthic agents
Antacids, laxatives, oils	Magnesium hydroxide
Enemas	Water, soap solution, irritants, hypertonic salt solutions

pass trophozoites containing red blood cells in their stools. Such patients are therapeutic challenges as ulcerative colitis may require steroids, drugs that can be disastrous for patients with invasive amebic dysentery. In these circumstances, amebic serology can be a considerable help. Indirect fluorescent antibody and various agglutination procedures offer sensitive screening techniques, while gel diffusion and cellulose acetate precipitation tests are highly specific. A positive test strongly suggests a diagnosis of amebiasis. Fecal antigen detection tests are now commercially available, and colorimetric polymerase chain reaction (PCR) techniques have high specificity and sensitivity.

Treatment

One of the current standard therapies for both intestinal and extra-intestinal amebiasis is metronidazole (Flagyl), 250 mg 3 times daily for 10 days. Higher doses and longer regimens may be necessary. It can be an unpleasant drug to take, sometimes causing nausea and vomiting. It leaves a bitter taste in the mouth. The patient must be warned that the urine can become discolored and that he or she may have an allergic reaction to alcohol during the course of treatment. Clinical and epidemiological experience will sometimes demand an alternate therapy. A combination of paromomycin (Humatin) 250 mg TID and doxycycline

(50 mg BID), for 10 days, is another effective regimen. The combination is also useful in treating those who cannot tolerate metronidazole. Diloxanide furoate is a safe and effective luminal amebicide (500 mg orally 3 times daily for 10 days). Severely ill patients may require rehydration and/or blood transfusion; and in this group, a preliminary 3 to 5 day course of doxycycline should be given before proceeding to metronidazole or alternative therapy. It should also be noted that a half-dozen other amebicidal compounds and combinations of drugs are available for the occasional patient who does not respond to, or cannot tolerate, the therapies cited here.

Other Gastrointestinal Manifestations of Amebiasis

Chronic localized granulomatous masses may form in the bowel wall. In the appendiceal and cecal area, they may cause intestinal obstruction and require differentiation from tuberculosis, carcinoma, and actinomycosis. A barium enema may reveal a cone-shaped cecum. Large, fixed lesions on the mucosa of the large bowel, amebomas, may closely resemble colon carcinoma. The barium enema may show a typical "apple core" deformity tapering at one end. In such cases, surgery should be avoided, if possible, until the effect of metronidazole or entamide furoate is seen. Intestinal amebiasis may also cause rectal ulceration with fistulae formation, which may be further complicated by amebic involvement of the perianal and surrounding skin. Severe cutaneous and subcutaneous ulceration may follow, and similar lesions may occur on the abdominal wall following surgery.

In asymptomatic individuals, treatment is not indicated when *E. histolytica/E. dispar* has been detected, but *E. histolytica* has not been identified, and serology is negative. In endemic areas, as much as 80% of the healthy population may be passing *E. dispar*. In nonendemic areas, passers of cysts originating from invasive forms of *E. histolytica* can be identified by history and clinical examination, by positive serology or antigen detection. These patients should be treated. Treatment can be with diloxanide furoate 500 mg 3 times daily for 10 days, or with paromomycin or metronidazole, both for 250 mg 3 times daily for the same duration.

Amebic Liver Abscess

Pathology

Entamoeba histolytica species that have invaded the colonic mucosa may be carried to the liver where they can multiply and produce a necrotic lesion or lesions with liquefaction of liver cells resulting in an amebic liver abscess. The contents of these abscesses does not consist of pus, and on ordinary media, it is sterile. Typically, the fluid is said to resemble anchovy paste sauce, but may be quite pale in color, and ameba are seldom found, being confined to the growing wall of the lesion. In 53% of cases, the abscess is in the right lobe of the liver; in 8% in the left lobe; and in 25%, both lobes are affected.

Clinical Features

The usual presentation of an amebic liver abscess is with a high swinging fever, pain in the right hypochondrium, sometimes radiating to the right shoulder. The liver is felt to be enlarged and is extremely tender on palpation. There is a moderate neutrophilic leukocytosis, and the chest x-ray may reveal elevation of the right diaphragm. The diagnosis of hepatic amebiasis should be strongly considered in patients with this constellation of symptoms and findings, especially if they are in or have come from an endemic area.

Other patients with amebic hepatic abscess may present with acute pleuritic pain, cough, sputum, and fever, and physical examination reveals abnormal signs at the right lung base. A chest x-ray may show shadowing in the right lower lobe with or without a pleural effusion; it is not surprising that such patients are occasionally referred to consultants as suffering from antibiotic resistant pneumonia. Other patients display the symptoms and signs of a pericardial effusion. Perhaps the most confusing presentation is seen in patients with a chronic amebic liver abscess, for these patients have neither fever nor leukocytosis. They may complain of vague upper abdominal pain or discomfort, anorexia, severe weight loss, and general ill health. The liver is found to be enlarged, hard, and often irregular, but not tender. A common misdiagnosis is that of secondary carcinoma, and this may prove to be erroneous only on the autopsy table.

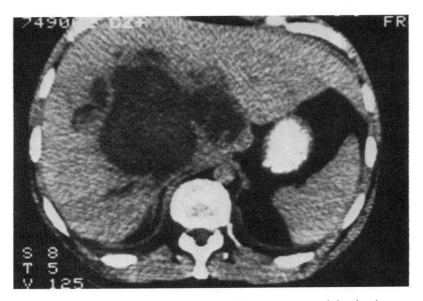

FIGURE 14: Computerized tomography (CT) scan demonstrating a multiloculated amebic abscess.

Patients with amebic abscess of the liver may seek medical care only years after leaving an endemic area, and commonly there is no history suggestive of past amebic liver abscess. Stool studies are frequently negative for ova and parasites. Until recently, one could expect little help from the laboratory. Now, if facilities are available, ultrasound will reveal a well encapsulated intrahepatic lesion or lesions with multiple, evenly distributed echoes that are weaker than those from a tumor but more numerous than those evoked by a hydatid cyst. Computerized tomography (CT scan) or magnetic resonance imaging (MRI) can also offer a visual picture of the abscess defects, as can ultrasound. Serological techniques will almost always demonstrate specific serum antibodies.

However, in many endemic tropical situations, facilities are simply not available for ultrasound, MRI, or CT studies, and the significance of the presence or magnitude of antibodies in the serum is questionable. In these circumstances, the diagnosis is still best confirmed by the rapid and characteristic response to treatment with metronidazole, or in the case of a chronic abscess, by aspiration after chemotherapy coverage has begun. Other conditions that simulate hepatic amebiasis include pyogenic abscesses, abscess associated with flukes, infective hydatid cysts, and primary hepatoma.

Treatment

Most amebic liver abscesses respond well to metronidazole 800 mg 3 times daily for 10 days or tinidazole 2 g daily for 6 days. These drugs may be supplemented by chloroquine diphosphate 300 mg base daily for 15 days. A luminal amebicide, diloxanide furoate, must complete the treatment schedule.

In the majority of patients, there is very obvious improvement within 48 to 72 hours, but in some cases, relapse occurs while they are still on treatment. In these patients, aspiration of the abscess should be undertaken without delay and may have to be repeated. Open surgical drainage should be avoided, if at all possible. CT, MRI, and ultrasound defects will remain for many months after clinical improvement.

Amebic abscesses may also occur in the lung and closely resemble pyogenic lung abscesses. Trophozoites may be detected in blood-stained sputum. Abscesses in the spleen and brain may also follow hematogenous dissemination.

Prevention

Amebiasis flourishes wherever sanitation is poor. Control is possible only after improvement in basic community hygiene through the use of properly constructed latrines, the provision of satisfactory water supply systems, and the elimination of the use of fresh "night soil" as a fertilizer. Travelers to the tropics should be warned against eating uncooked vegetables and unpeeled fruit as well as the danger of drinking unboiled or untreated water. So-called intestinal medicaments taken as prophylactics are ineffective and indeed add diagnostic difficulties. Household spread can be interrupted by educating contacts regarding the importance of hand-washing after contact with potentially infected feces; for example, a mother may become infected from a young child because the mother is changing the child's underwear or diaper and rarely pauses to wash hands. Sexual partners also rarely get up to wash hands, and oral sexual activity obviously increases the risk of contamination.

Bacterial and Rickettsial Diseases

Typhoid Fever

Typhoid occurs worldwide but is much more prevalent in the tropics and subtropics. Typhoid and malaria are the two most common causes of fever in persons recently returned from a visit abroad. More than 90% of patients with typhoid in developed countries are infections imported from the tropics.

The Organism

Salmonella typhi is a gram negative, motile, rod-shaped bacteria with a flagellum. Unlike *E. coli*, which has a similar appearance, it does not ferment lactose. Tryptic broth or 10% Oxgall are used for culturing the organism from the blood, and selective *Salmonella-Shigella* medium (SS) is employed in culturing feces. After infection, antibodies are raised against three antigens: a somatic o lipopolysaccharide antigen, a flagellar H protein antigen, and a capsular Vi polysaccharide antigen.

Pathology

Infection is acquired by the ingestion of an adequate number of *S. typhi*, the chance of acquiring clinical typhoid being directly related to the number of organisms. Common vehicles of infection are contaminated water, milk, and food. Hypochlorhydric persons are at greater risk.

The organisms penetrate small intestinal mucosal cells (the microfold or M cells), which overlie lymphatic aggregations (Peyer's patches). They then multiply within the mononuclear cells of these aggregates and in related mesenteric lymph nodes. At a critical point, sufficient organisms are released into the blood to cause a bacteremia, and this coincides with the end of the incubation period. *S. typhi* are then carried to various tissues, especially of the liver, spleen, and lymph nodes, where they further multiply in macrophages. The gall bladder is invaded, and *S. typhi* reappear in the intestine and penetrate the mucosa. Hyperplasia within Peyer's patches of the ileum may be followed by necrosis and sloughing. The resulting ulcers are found in the long axis of the bowel along the antimesenteric border.

Hemorrhage and/or perforation may follow. There may be cloudy swelling and focal necrosis of hepatocytes; the spleen becomes enlarged, soft, and congested. Metastatic foci of infection may lead to abscess formation throughout the body. If the patient survives, eventual healing is usually complete without scarring.

Clinical Features

Incubation periods of 3 to 60 days have been reported but the average is 8 to 18 days. In "typical typhoid," there is a step-like rise in temperature during the first week to 102°F to 104°F, accompanied by pronounced headache, malaise, and anorexia. Other symptoms include a sore throat, a dry cough, epistaxis, vague abdominal discomfort, and, frequently, constipation. The tongue is coated, and the pharynx may appear dry and inflamed. There is a relative bradycardia, especially when related to the temperature, and a relative leukopenia.

During the second week, the temperature remains high, but now the pulse rate catches up. Abdominal symptoms become more definite, and there may be pain and tenderness in the right iliac fossa. The liver is often felt 2 to 3 cm below the costal margin, and the spleen becomes palpable as a soft, tender mass just below the left costal margin. Raised pink 2 to 5 mm macules (rose spots), which fade on pressure, occur in crops on the trunk. Toward the end of the second week and into the third week, the patient enters the most dangerous phase of the illness. Constipation may give place to "pea soup diarrhea." A toxic encephalopathy may develop, the patient becoming confused or obtunded, lying immobile in bed, staring blankly although still rousable; other patients show agitation, disorientation, and delirium. Headache remains severe and may prevent sleep; meningismus is not uncommon. It is at this stage that hemorrhage and perforation most commonly occur.

However, typhoid is more often "atypical" than "typical." The fever may be high, low, or intermittent. The relative bradycardia is quite inconstant, and rose spots may be absent and are almost never found in those with dark skins. As in many fevers, dysuria is not uncommon and the white blood cell (WBC) may vary from 1,200 to 22,000 per mm³. Typhoid in young children may be particularly "atypical," commonly presenting with severe diarrhea, vomiting, dehydration, meningismus, and convulsions. While most pediatric typhoid cases will have a significant fever, even this feature may be missing in severely malnourished children and in those with profound anemia. Jaundice, which is only occasionally seen in adults, occurs in about 7% of children.

Another situation in which diagnostic skill is required is defining when a perforation has occurred. It may occur even after a patient has begun to respond to antibiotic treatment; daily, careful examination of the abdomen is mandatory. Indications include the onset of abdominal pain; tenderness and guarding, especially in the right iliac fossa; vomiting; an increase in pulse rate with a fall in the fever; abdominal distension with or without free fluid; and absent bowel sounds. The differentiation from intestinal ileus, another complication of typhoid, is particularly difficult. Gas under the diaphragm can be demonstrated by x-ray in about 75% of patients who have perforated. In the tropics, many patients with typhoid remain ambulant and may present at hospital only for the first time when a febrile illness, with or without diarrhea, is complicated by the acute abdominal pain of perforation.

Intestinal hemorrhage is another serious complication, and the bleeding may be slight or profuse, the blood usually being bright red. Other complications include intestinal ileus; cholecystitis; hepatitis; suppurative parotitis; pneumonia; meningitis; endocarditis; peripheral neuritis; temporary nerve deafness; femoral thrombosis; and osteomyelitis affecting the lumbar sacral spine, ribs, or long bones. Focal inflammatory lesions, such as a splenic abscess, may occur.

Diagnosis

Isolation of S. typhi is the only unequivocal method of confirming the diagnosis, and this is best sought by culture of whole blood; other sources include feces, urine, duodenal, and bone marrow aspirates. Cultures are usually positive during the final week of the illness. The main difficulty with diagnostic cultures is that growth may be delayed and that adequate facilities are often unavailable where typhoid is most common. In these circumstances, the much-reviled Widal reaction can be a considerable help. A titer of 1:80 of the 0 antibody is present in about 70% of proven typhoids and is negative in controls. The results are available within 24 hours. The H antigen may be elevated from previous typhoid inoculations. Newer diagnostic techniques include an ELISA test using Vi antigen that are most useful as epidemiologic tools and for screening food handlers.

Treatment

S. typhi are sensitive to many antibiotics. Effective antimicrobials include ampicillin, amoxicillin, and trimethoprim sulphamethoxazole. Excellent results have recently been reported in multiresistant infections treated with oral ciprofloxacin. Chloramphenicol is an effective remedy in a dose of 50 mg per kg bw in 4 divided doses daily for 14 days. The fever may not subside for 5 to 7 days, and blood cultures may remain positive for 10 days. Plasmid-borne resistance to chloramphenicol does occur. The hematologic side effects of chloramphenicol are also well known, and careful follow-up is always indicated. In seriously ill patients, dexamethazone is a valuable adjunct.

For many years, the approach advised for perforation was intestinal aspiration, intravenous fluids, and parenteral chloramphenicol, but this regimen carried a very high mortality, and opinion has now swung firmly in favor of surgical intervention. Laparotomy should be preceded by general measures, including decompression of the gastrointestinal tract via nasogastric tube; rehydration; transfusion, if necessary; and intravenous (IV) therapy with chloramphenicol and amoxicillin. Depending on the state of the bowel, operations may consist of simple closure or excision. In patients in whom perforation has occurred more than 3 days before admission, IV methyl prednisolone succinate given 6 hourly for 6 to 8 doses is said to improve results. The mortality following surgical treatment has now been reduced to 10%.

Whatever treatment is provided, relapse may be expected in 5% to 15% of patients. This usually occurs about 11 days after cessation of chemotherapy, and the relapse is usually less severe than the original attack. Two or three relapses have been reported. Furthermore, approximately 10% of patients will continue to excrete *S. typhi* in their stools for some months and 3% for more than one year, the latter being defined as chronic carriers. Treatment of these chronic carriers remains unsatisfactory; the latest recommendations are ampicillin or amoxicillin plus probenecid daily for 3 months; or, alternatively, trimethoprim sulphamethoxazole daily for the same period. Some patients will respond only after cholecystectomy.

Epidemiology

The source of infection is ultimately the feces of patients with typhoid or the feces or urine of carriers. The incidence of carriers is particularly high in regions with a high prevalence of liver and blood fluke infection as *S. typhi* colonizes the tegmentum of these parasites.

S. typhi persists for several weeks in water, ice, dust, and dried sewage as well as on clothing. It survives and multiplies in food and seafood, such as oysters and mussels grown in polluted waters. Food may be contaminated through the hands of carriers, and in hot, dry climates, the "filthy feet of fecal feeding flies" are important methods of transmission. The state of many wells and water holes in parts of Africa must account for much of the high prevalence of this disease.

Prevention

The key to prevention lies in adequate sewage disposal and the provision of protected water supplies, but universal safe water is unlikely to be realized for some time. Meanwhile, there is a need for a cheap, effective, safe, and practical vaccine for mass immunization of children. Vaccines in use and those under trial include the following:

> Heat/phenol inactivated whole cell vaccine: This is the only vaccine available in much of the tropical world and provides 50% to 65% protection. It has to be given parenterally in 2 doses but produces

unpleasant local and systemic effects because of the presence of an endotoxin. Booster doses are required every 3 years.

Acetone inactivated whole cell vaccine: This is given in the same manner, but due to the preservation of the Vi antigen, it provides about 80% protection. However, it also contains endotoxin, is expensive, and is generally unavailable in the tropics.

Vi antigen polysaccharide vaccine: This Vi antigen vaccine is prepared by detergent extraction, and is free of contaminating endotoxin. It is given as a single intramuscular injection.

Ty 21: This oral live vaccine seemed a promising development, but 4 doses are currently required, and side effects are common.

Other Tropical Bacterial Fevers

Diagnosis and treatment of fevers constitute much of the practice of tropical medicine. Protozoal causes have already been described. In addition, a number of fevers, besides typhoid, are caused by bacterial infections. Because a group of them share so many features, it is convenient to consider them together.

Common clinical presentations are fever, chills, headache, cough, lassitude, anorexia, vomiting, and generalized pains. Most typhoid patients have, as a physical feature, splenomegaly. Routine laboratory tests often provide little help in diagnosis, and confirmation is often possible only during convalescence. Most are zoonoses, and all are closely connected with a particular geographical environment, so that a history of exposure can be very helpful.

In the subtropical environments of the Mediterranean, the Middle East, and into east Africa, the following bacterial infections are endemic.

Brucellosis

Brucella melitensis causes chronic mastitis and contagious abortion in goats, sheep, and camels. The main source of human infection is unpasteurized goat's milk and its products. The epidemiology and bacteriology of the disease were defined by David Bruce in a series of classic studies on the island of Malta where thousands of British soldiers had been infected after obtaining local milk supplies. *Brucella* is a small, nonmotile, gram-negative coccobacillus that is difficult to grow. Special media is required in an atmosphere of 10% carbon dioxide; even then, growth may be very slow. It is an obligate intracellular organism that elicits a granuloma reaction.

Clinical Features

The acute stage, lasting 2 to 3 weeks, is characterized by late afternoon fever spikes to 104F, associated with shaking chills and followed by severe sweating, often giving off a peculiar sour odor. Patients tend to be particularly miserable with severe headaches and depression. Monoarticular arthritis involving large joints is often a prominent feature, and orchitis also occurs. A rare fulminant form of brucellosis has also been described.

Sequelae include a subacute form of the disease with "undulant fever," resembling the Pel Epstein temperature curve of lymphoma, involvement of the sacroiliac and intervertebral joints, and sometimes bacterial endocarditis. A chronic form is recognized in east Africa, which closely resembles kala azar with hepatomegaly and hypersplenism.

The initial diagnosis of acute brucellosis often must be made on clinical grounds; a history of exposure is, obviously, very helpful. The diagnosis may be confirmed by a positive agglutination reaction, or, preferably, by a rising titer of IgM antibody by ELISA. Blood cultures may prove positive, but results are often delayed.

Most patients respond to treatment with doxycycline for 4 to 12 weeks; patients who relapse, or who suffer from more serious manifestations, may require concomitant cotrimoxazole or streptomycin. Gentamycin, and rifampicin are used in patients with endocarditis. *Brucella abortus*, *B. suis*, and *B. canis*, with cattle, pigs, and dogs as the primary reservoirs of infection, can cause similar illnesses in man.

Q Fever

Coxiella burneti, a rickettsia-like organism, also infects the female genital organs and mammary glands of goats, sheep, and cattle in the same regions where brucellosis flourishes. Infection in local children is mainly acquired from unpasteurized milk. The hardy *Coxiella* organisms are also present in the uterine discharges of parturition and are spread in contaminated dust inhaled by nonimmune adult visitors.

Patients may complain of sore throat, conjunctival injection, and cough. While patients with brucellosis may occasionally show pulmonary infiltration, this is an almost constant finding in Q fever, appearing as single or multiple soft shadows, usually in the lower lobes. There may be evidence of a mild hepatitis.

The illness usually subsides spontaneously after 1 to 3 weeks, but in some patients, organisms persist in the body in a dormant state, only to emerge later to cause myocarditis, meningoencephalitis, epididymitis, spinal osteomyelitis, or bacterial endocarditis. A diagnosis is confirmed by a rising titer of serum antibodies to Phase 2 antigen; in chronic infection, there is a high titer of Phase 1 antibodies. Other serologic tests are also available.

Treatment is with doxycycline or chloramphenicol. Although drug therapy will not hasten the usual spontaneous recovery, it is believed that it may prevent persisting infection.

Tick Typhus

Mild forms of spotted fever—tick typhus—occur in Africa and along the Mediterranean coast. The etiologic organism is *Rickettsia conori*, and the vectors are hard ticks of the *Ixodidae* family. Transovarial infection occurs in the tick, so it serves as both a vector and a reservoir of infection. As in other forms of typhus, the basic pathological lesions involve the endothelium of the smaller blood vessels.

The principal diagnostic features are the presence of an eschar; the appearance on the fifth day of a centripetal, maculopapular, sometimes petechial rash; and also signs of encephalitis. OXK and OX19 serologic titers may be elevated. The encephalitis is often rather mild, usually manifest by only a certain dullness of response. In severe cases, there may be stupor and confusion. There may also be evidence of facial and conjunctival congestion and a mild hepatitis. The diagnosis is usually clear from the clinical features and is confirmed by a rising titer of specific antibodies. Patients respond well to doxycycline or chloramphenicol.

Scrub Typhus

The most common acute fever requiring admission to hospital in rural Malaysia is scrub typhus. The causative organism is *Rickettsia tsutsugamushi*, primarily infecting rodents and transmitted by larval mites *Trombicula deliense* or *Trombicula akamushi*, in which transovarial transmission also occurs. The mites, which live in the soil, require only one blood feed during a life cycle involving larval, nymph, and adult stages, and this is taken in the first larval stage. The "jiggers" climb on to the long "lalang grass" to await the passage of rats, but will also attack man. Infection is prevalent in many rural areas but may be very localized; particularly dangerous sites are palm oil plantations. Scrub typhus can be acquired in any place where rats and mites coexist; in the cities of southeast Asia, it is known as "back garden disease."

Clinical Features

Clinical features are similar to those seen in tick typhus but tend to be more severe, especially in patients older than 40. The rash is centrifugal rather than centripetal. The encephalitis is often manifest by dullness or stupor by day and excitement at night. For some unknown reason, eschars—common in European and Japanese patients—are seldom found in Malays and Indians, in whom the rash may also be difficult to discern.

The diagnosis must initially be based only on clinical grounds and is more difficult in the absence of an eschar and rash. It may be confirmed during convalescence by demonstrating a rising indirect immunologic antibody titer to a trivalent antigen. A modification of the Weil Felix reaction using the OXK strain of *Bacillus proteus* is also used as an auxiliary test. No attempt should be made to isolate the organism except in special centers.

Treatment with doxycycline is effective, but in patients in whom there is doubt as to whether the illness is typhus or typhoid, chloramphenicol is often preferred. Preventive programs based on residual insecticides are important in endemic areas. Individual traveler's can be protected by a single weekly dose of doxycycline (200 mg) taken while in an infected zone and for 2 weeks thereafter.

Murine (shop) typhus is endemic in southeast Asia. It is an urban infection with *Rickettsia typhi*, primarily involving domestic rats and transmitted by the oriental rat flea, *Xenopsylla cheopis*. The illness is clinically indistinguishable from scrub typhus, but this matters little as the treatment is the same. It can be distinguished during convalescence by the demonstration of specific antibody.

Louse-borne typhus caused by *Rickettsia prowazeki* occurs in highland areas of the tropics but is primarily a disease of cold climate (e.g., the Balkans) and becomes epidemic in the overcrowded refugee camps of war-torn areas. It presents with petechial rashes, and in 50% of cases, meningoencephalitis develops. Treatment with chloramphenicol or doxycycline is effective. Delousing and prophylactic therapy with doxycycline is indicated in endemic situations.

Tick-borne Relapsing Fever

Various strains of *Borrelia* infect rodents in the tropics. They are transmitted to men by soft ticks, which gather in large numbers in caves and other sheltered places. This has long been known to the Bedouins; before taking shelter themselves in caves, they drive their goats and sheep in first so that the ticks become satisfied with an animal blood meal. In Africa, the tick vectors have become domesticated, living under shady trees or in the mud walls and floors of village huts, and feeding only on man. *Borrelia* are spirochetes and are seen in blood films as corkscrewed, motile organisms with 5 to 10 regular spirals. Like trypanosomes, they have the capacity to change surface antigens when challenged by antibodies, so that repeated attacks of fever lasting 3 to 4 days are separated by apyrexial intervals of 7 to 10 days.

There is a tendency to facial and conjunctival congestion, and both headache and muscle pains may be severe. Aseptic meningitis, seventh cranial nerve palsy, and iridocyclitis have been frequently reported. There may also be evidence of a mild hepatitis, but the most characteristic feature is the temperature chart: a high fever falling abruptly to normal on the third or fourth day only to recur after 7 to 10 days. Sequelae are uncommon in the Mediterranean area, but fulminant, fatal cases still occur in east Africa.

Diagnosis depends on identifying the etiologic spirochetes in thick and thin blood films Giemsa or Leishman stains. Treatment is with doxycycline, but if this is started during a period of high bacteremia, it may be followed by a severe reaction. Prevention is accomplished by avoiding ticks, wearing protective clothing, and using insecticides.

Plague

Although the clinical course of plague is as fulminant today as when pandemics of the disease decimated the world, it is more a potential than an actual health hazard. Fewer than 1,500 cases are reported annually to WHO, the majority from endemic foci in northern Peru and central India. However, because it is an extremely widespread enzootic disease, plague is poised constantly on a delicate balance, and when man and domestic rats contact the wild rodent reservoirs, human infection occurs. Plague is also recognized as a potential bioterrorist agent.

Rodent fleas, of which the most important is *Xenopsylla cheopis*, ingest *Pasturella pestis* from infected rats. The organisms multiply in the esophagus, or proventriculus, of the flea to such an extent that they cause blockage or impaction. As the thirsty flea sucks a second blood meal, it regurgitates bacilli into the wound site. Although wild rodents tolerate infection well—and, therefore, are excellent reservoirs—domestic rats react in much the same way as man does. When they die, their fleas seek another source of food, and man enters the infective cycle.

Sporadic cases that illustrate this epidemiologic cycle are reported, for example, in the southwestern United States, and devastating epidemics still occur in areas where man cohabitates closely with infected rats or when man to man transmission of pneumonic plague is not controlled. Camus' tale of one such epidemic in Oran is both a literary classic and a fine medical description.

Pasturella pestis, the causative organism of plague, is a gram-negative, nonmotile coccobacillus found in the sputum of pneumonic victims and in enlarged lymph nodes, or buboes, the spleen, and the heart of bubonic plague patients. The virulence of *P. pestis* depends on the presence of somatic (V or W) antigens, and a protective, surface antigen (F-I) and the production of a necrotizing endotoxin. The bacilli multiply in lymph nodes and disseminate only after toxic damage to neighboring vascular beds permits spread via the bloodstream. Diffuse hemorrhage is common in the epicardium, pericardium, spleen, liver, kidney, and brain. In victims of pneumonic plague, pulmonary and pleural hemorrhages are prominent.

The incubation period of human plague averages 3 to 5 days, but symptoms may be seen in primary pneumonic patients within 24 hours after infection. In all types, the onset is acute, with fever, chills, confusion and prostration. In the pneumonic form of the disease, cyanosis and coma are common; in bubonic plague, painful, tender, and occasionally, ulcerating inguinal and cervical adenopathy is characteristic. In overwhelming septicemic plague, the victim may die before any signs are evident.

During an epidemic, the presence of dying rats and contact cases make confident clinical diagnosis possible. Laboratory confirmation in sporadic cases is essential. The organism can be visualized in gram or methylene blue preparations from buboes, sputum, or blood in the living and from autopsy material of humans, fleas, or rodents. Culture on selective media enhances isolation. Thermoprecipitin and fluorescent antibody tests are also available.

Treatment in all types of plague is effective if it is given early in the disease; plague is usually fatal if therapy is delayed. Combinations of chloramphenicol, streptomycin, and tetracyclines are recommended. Except as a potential bioterrorist threat, the temperate climate physician's concern with plague will be limited largely to advice for travelers in regard to prophylaxis. An inactivated vaccine is available but produces significant side effects, and is only partially effective. It must be repeated every 6 months. Only those persons who expect to be in contact with patients who are known to be infected or with infected animals should be advised to undergo inoculation. No nation currently requires plague vaccination for visitors. If contact is expected, prophylactic use of tetracycline is advisable.

Anthrax

Once a common occupational disease among wool sorters and tanners in Europe and the United States, anthrax remains endemic in the Middle East, Africa, and India. Because of the resistant quality and survival of anthrax spores, the disease is now of major concern because of its potential use as a biologic terrorist weapon.

The aerobic gram-positive organisms (first described by Koch in 1877) produce spores that can withstand extreme heats and remain alive for decades. The spores germinate producing toxins that, in an infected site, alters local vascular permeability assuring rapid spread to local nodes where hemorrhage and massive edema occur. Typical cutaneous lesions range from a local necrotic pustule to extreme ulcerative and edematous lesions of the face, neck, and arms. Inhalation of spores can result in pulmonary hemorrhage with gross hilar adenopathy and rapidly extend to a fatal septicemia and meningitis.

Diagnosis is usually based on a history of geographic or occupational exposure. The organism can be readily cultured from skin lesions, but one should avoid incisions or biopsies because iatrogenic spread is likely. Organisms can also be isolated from the sputum of pulmonary anthrax victims, but that is most often a postmortem finding. Treatment is with IV or intramuscular (IM) penicillin, doxycycline, or ciprofloxin. A vaccine is available and was used, because of the fear of biologic attack, in the Iraq and Afghanistan wars. The efficacy and safety of the vaccine are acceptable, but mass public prophylaxis has not been undertaken due to significant side effects.

Leptospirosis

The common bacterial fevers of the warm, moist, tropical lands of southeast Asia differ from those of the Mediterranean and Middle East. Typhoid is common in both regions, but brucellosis and Q fever are not seen; tick typhus is replaced by scrub typhus, and relapsing fever by leptospirosis.

More than 40 strains of pathogenic leptospires have been identified in Malaysia, so it is not surprising that this infection is common; it accounts for more than 10% of hospital admissions for fever in rural areas. In neighboring Thailand, serologic surveys show that 27% of the population have had previous infection with leptospirosis. The etiologic organism is a spirochete, *Leptospira interrogans*, which primarily infects rats; this animal host is unaffected but excretes vast numbers of leptospires in the urine. The subspecies that causes classical Weil's Disease is *Leptospira icterohaemorragiae*, with the name providing an apt description of the problems caused. The near-impenetrable mountain jungles of southeast Asia abound with rats that, like humans, find the banks of streams easy pathways. There rats deposit their leptospires, which are then carried down by tropical rain storms to the rice fields below and come in contact with bare-legged workers. They enter the body through abrasions in the skin. Leptospires can survive long periods in fresh water or mud. Domestic animals, cattle, and swine can also become infected and serve as an added link in the chain of transmission from rodents to humans.

Clinical Features

The infected victim presents with a high fever, congested face, and suffused eyes. Patients suffer intensely from muscle pain, so much so that squeezing a calf muscle is liable to be followed by a violent reaction. Prostration may seem to be out of proportion to the vital signs. Abdominal pain, tenderness, and vomiting associated with a mild neutrophilic leukocytosis may prompt the misdiagnosis of acute appendicitis. Complications include a bleeding tendency and acute renal failure, but in contrast with Weil's disease in Europe and America, jaundice is uncommon. Bleeding into the lung can cause hemoptysis, and soft infiltrates are seen in chest x-ray.

In addition to raised neutrophils, one often finds a thrombocytopenia. The urine contains protein, blood, and casts. The blood urea may be slightly raised. Any doubt as to the diagnosis is quickly dispelled by a therapeutic trial of penicillin. This causes a dramatic fall in the temperature, sometimes accompanied by collapse. The sensitized erythrocyte lysis test of Meers and Ringrose is commonly used to support the diagnosis, but identification of the serological strain of the infecting leptospires requires specialist facilities. In contrast with the *Borrelia* of relapsing fever, leptospires are found in blood only in the early phase, and in the urine in later stages.

Treatment with penicillin is usually preferred, but doxycycline or tetracycline can be employed in the penicillin allergic patient. Because of the multiplicity of strains and the ability of the organism to survive long periods in water, public health measures have been unsuccessful. Individual protection can be provided by a weekly doxycycline dose.

Melioidosis

Burkholderia pseudomallei is another gram-negative, motile, flagellated bacillus that abounds in the warm, moist soil and surface waters of Malaysia, Vietnam, Thailand, and northern Australia. Infection is thought to be usually acquired percutaneously through skin abrasions. It was once, erroneously, considered a rare infection limited to tramps, alcoholics, and drug addicts. Antibodies are demonstrated in as many as 85% of some indigenous rural populations in northern Thailand, and this infection accounts in the region for 2.5% of patients admitted to hospital with fever.

Clinical Features

The clinical manifestations depend greatly on the immunologic state of the individual infected, and signs and symptoms can be so varied that the diagnosis is often missed.

  Asymptomatic seroconversion is probably the most common result of infection in local children, but the organisms may persist in a dormant state only to cause serious disease years later when immunity is compromised for one reason or another.
  A single subcutaneous abscess that may be suppurative for months or progress to localized granulomatous lesions in lymph nodes, joints, and the liver.
  A short-term fever that may resolve spontaneously, but in vulnerable patients, progresses to a fulminant hyperpyrexia with shaking chills and severe diarrhea.
  A pneumonia with an x-ray appearance of upper lobe infiltrates with or without cavitation. The radiographic picture can be easily misdiagnosed as pulmonary tuberculosis.
  Septicemia with rigors, high fever, prostration, diarrhea, and multiple abscess formation rapidly leading to death.
  Chronic granulomatous inflammation in lymph nodes, bone, joints, liver, and elsewhere.

The diagnosis is difficult because of the ubiquitous nature of the infection, and even a serum antibody titer of 1:80 cannot be taken as evidence of active infection. It is, therefore, all the more important to isolate the organism but this requires informing the laboratory of its suspected presence. Otherwise, the organisms are likely to be merely labeled as coliforms. The appearance of colonies is characteristic. Treatment of the less-serious manifestations can be with augmentin or a prolonged course of doxycycline.

Bartonellosis.

This strange disease is endemic along the steep valley slopes of Peru, Columbia, and Ecuador within well delineated limits of climate and altitude. It may present as a rapidly fatal, febrile anemia, as a chronic dermatological disease, or as both.

The etiological organism, *Bartonella bacilliformis*, is transmitted from man to man by the bite of an infected *Phlebotomus* sandfly, *Lutzomia verrucarim*. After an incubation period varying from 2 to 3 weeks, acute symptoms may appear; most prominent are generalized pains in muscles and joints, tender enlargement of lymph nodes, fever, and a sudden hemolytic anemia.

The liver and spleen enlarge. This phase of bartonellosis is called "Oroya fever" or "Carrion's disease" (named after the young medical student who died of the infection while studying it). It usually lasts 1 to 2 months and is diagnosed by visualizing *B. bacilliformis* within peripheral red blood cells. If untreated, the fatality rate varies from 10% to 40%. There is an excellent response to treatment with chloramphenicol.

Irrespective of whether the patient has suffered an attack of Oroya fever or not, the second phase of the illness may develop 4 months after infection. This consists of a generalized hemangiomatous dermal eruption, verruga peruana. Verrugas formed by proliferating endothelial cells and newly formed capillaries appear as flattened or pedunculated vascular nodules mainly on the face and extensor aspects of the limbs. They also develop in the upper gastrointestinal tract and female genitalia, where they may cause bleeding. Larger nodules, growing to the size of pigeon eggs, may be found on the knees and elbows. The lesions may persist for several years. Although there is no successful treatment for the verruga stage, the prognosis is good, and one attack will provide a lasting immunity.

Tuberculosis

As the twenty-first century begins, tuberculosis (TB) remains a global scourge. In fact, the incidence and severity of tuberculosis, especially in the tropics, is rising. The United Nations estimates that more than 9 million people are infected with TB, with an <10% prevalence of HIV in new adult cases. In Africa, south of the Sahara, tuberculosis patients have a mortality rate 25 times higher than those recorded in the Americas. Dual infection with HIV and TB, compounded by polyparasitic infections, malnutrition, and emerging multi-drug resistant strains of *Mycobacterium tuberculosis* are a lethal combination. In a broad swath across southeast Asia from India through Bangladesh, Myanmar, Indonesia, and Thailand, TB is the leading cause of infectious deaths and the leading killer of women. In most European countries, and in the United States, almost 50% of new cases are in immigrants from developing nations, and the ever-increasing movement of large refugee populations accounts for the spread of TB in countries where control programs had largely contained transmission.

The etiologic agent of tuberculosis is an acid-fast (AFB) bacteria, *Mycobacterium tuberculosis*, and, occasionally, *Mycobacterium bovis* and *Mycobacterium africanum*. Infection typically occurs when bacilli are spread through air droplets when an individual with active pulmonary TB coughs. The droplets can remain suspended in the air for a prolonged period of time, especially in a dark environment. However, 5 minutes of direct sunlight will kill the bacilli.

After inhalation, *M. tuberculosis* bacilli multiply within lung tissue, forming a primary complex known as a "Ghon focus," usually associated with hilar lymphadenopathy. In the normal immunocompetent individual, the body mounts a significant hypersensitivity/cellular reaction against the primary complex to kill the bacilli and contain the infection. This usually occurs within 4 to 6 weeks of infection.

However, a few dormant bacilli may persist with the only evidence being a positive tuberculin skin test. In some individuals, the primary complex is not contained, and they may develop tuberculous pneumonia, which can be complicated by pleural effusions and collapse of lung tissue. Cervical lymphadenopathy, meningitis, pericarditis, hypersensitivity reactions (e.g., erythema nodosum), and miliary spread may also occur in uncontained primary infection.

Post-primary TB occurs when there is reactivation and/or reinfection with tubercle bacilli. Reactivation may be triggered by a weakening of the immune system (e.g., age, HIV, chemotherapy, other co-infections, malnutrition). In this setting, the immune reaction is localized and can be quite destructive. In the lungs, extensive damage and cavitation can occur, especially in the upper lobes. Pleural effusion, empyema, and pneumothorax are well-described complications. Extrapulmonary TB can potentially occur in any part of the body: hence the name, the "great imitator."

Clinical Features

The patient presenting with pulmonary TB often gives a history of fever, night sweats, weight loss, productive cough for greater than 2 to 3 weeks, dyspnea, and hemoptysis. Patients who are HIV-positive may have a nonclassic presentation.

TB meningitis is most commonly seen in infants and young children. It often presents with a more gradual onset than bacterial meningitis. Secondary to significant inflammatory reaction at the base of the brain, cranial nerve involvement is common, particularly of the optic and auditory nerves. Obstructive hydrocephalus may develop, leading to an increase in intracranial pressure. Spinal meningeal involvement may lead to paralysis. In infants, the initial presentation may be simply a failure to thrive. Diagnosis is made by lumbar puncture; a high opening pressure is present with white cells being predominantly lymphocytes, an elevated protein, and low glucose levels. A fibrin web may develop if the cerebrospinal fluid (CSF) is allowed to stand. The CSF should be examined for evidence of AFB and cultured if possible. A lumbar puncture should never be performed in a patient with evidence of raised intracranial pressure, seizures, or focal neurological findings. Tuberculomas may also develop, and present with symptoms consistent with an intracranial lesion. Diagnosis can be made with computerized tomography (CT) scan or MRI of the brain.

Tuberculous lymphadenitis occurs most commonly in the cervical region, but may present anywhere in the body. Initially, the nodes are firm and tender and then become fluctuant and matted together. Sinus tracts may develop as the lymph node undergoes necrosis. Diagnosis is made by biopsy of the lymph node. In a clinical setting of TB, biopsy may not be necessary.

In the tropics, TB is the most common cause for pericardial effusion. Patients present with chest pain, shortness of breath, and dizziness.

On physical exam hypotension, elevated jugular venous pressure, evidence of right sided heart failure, a pericardial rub, and distant heart sounds may be noted. Cardiac tamponade can develop.

Tuberculous involvement of the bone is also very common in the tropics, and if unrecognized/untreated, can result in devastating paralysis. The lower thoracic and lumbar regions of the spine are most commonly affected; however, it can occur anywhere. Patients usually present with chronic pain of the vertebral region involved, limitation of the movement, and sometimes, with an acute neurological finding. Diagnosis is made by plain films and biopsy/culture. Besides chemotherapy, surgical stabilization may be required.

Intestinal tuberculosis is most often associated with ingestion of *Mycobacterium bovis*. Peritoneal involvement occurs from post primary spread. Patients may have nonspecific abdominal complaints: weight loss, anorexia, abdominal pain, nausea, vomiting, and diarrhea. Intestinal obstruction may develop secondary to stricture formation. Ascites is common as the disease progresses. Diagnosis can occasionally be made by paracentesis, but peritoneal biopsy is usually required.

Tuberculous involvement of the kidneys can present with dysuria, nocturia, hematuria, flank pain, and less commonly, acute renal failure secondary to tuberculous interstitial nephritis. In males, chronic epidymitis or orchitis may develop. Female genital tract involvement presents with pelvic pain, possible vaginal bleeding, and infertility. On examination of the urine, a sterile pyuria is found. It is uncommon to find AFB in the urine. Cultivation of the *M. tuberculosis* confirms the diagnosis.

Infection of tuberculosis with HIV deserves special mention, especially in the tropics. Co-infection rapidly accelerates the disease process of both HIV and TB. It is important to remember that in HIV/AIDS patients, atypical presentations of TB frequently occur, and miliary disease is far more common. A high index of suspicion for simultaneous HIV infection needs to be held for all patients with TB.

Diagnosis

The standard assessment of a patient for pulmonary TB is to obtain, over a several-day period, three sets of sputum samples for microscopic examination. Chest physiotherapy can be performed to improve sputum production. A Ziehl-Neelsen stain can be used to look for evidence of acid-fast bacilli. Besides sputum, other clinical specimens may be examined: the contents of bronchoalveolar lavage, gastric lavage (an alternative in children who cannot produce sputum), pleural effusions, peritoneal and cerebrospinal fluid, lymph node biopsies, and bone marrow aspirates. The classic histological findings in a tissue biopsy are an area of centralized caseous necrosis surrounded by histiocytes, Langhans giant cells, and lymphocytes.

If facilities are available, the optimal diagnostic technique is to culture the bacilli. The usual culture medium is Lowenstein Jensen; however, liquid culture and automated systems can be used if available. *Mycobacterium tuberculosis* is very slow growing and may take as long as 8 weeks to develop a positive culture. Several molecular techniques using nucleic acid amplification have been developed. These tests are highly sensitive and specific, and several commercial kits are available. However, their use has been limited, by expense, to the developed world and major medical centers in the tropics.

Radiographic studies are also helpful in making a diagnosis of TB. Chest x-rays in post-primary TB often show apical/upper unilateral or bilateral infiltrates, cavitations, and calcifications. Pleural effusions can also be seen. Some patients (particularly HIV and immunocompromised) will have minimal changes or nonspecific findings on chest x-ray. Where CT scan of the chest is available, this may further help in evaluating a questionable chest x-ray.

The tuberculin skin test, developed from purified protein derived from the tubercle bacilli, relies on a hypersensitivity reaction that occurs 24 to 72 hours after intradermal inoculation. The test does not necessarily indicate active infection, only that a positive reacting individual has been exposed to the bacilli. The test may be negative in infected individuals who have the following conditions: malnutrition, severe infection, miliary TB, HIV, cancer, or other immunosuppressive conditions. A test is considered negative in a normal immunocompetent individual if the induration measures less than 10 mm after 48 to 72 hours. In a child who has received the BCG vaccine, up to 15 mm is considered negative.

Treatment

The cornerstone of successful TB treatment is patient compliance; this is best achieved by directly observed therapy (DOT). This approach is especially important in the tropics where nonadherence to drug regimens is, for many logistical reasons, a significant problem. Direct observation of the patient swallowing prescribed tablets has been successfully accomplished by a wide variety of personnel, ranging from trained health care workers to religious and community volunteers. Where a DOT program is in place, drug resistance decreases, and initial therapeutic responses of 75% to 90% are demonstrated in many tropical countries. Relapse rates are also dramatically lower. Treatment usually is based on several agents for synergism and to decrease drug resistance. Combinations of isoniazid, rifampin, ethambutol, pyrezinamide, thiacetazone, and the old standby, streptomycin, are among the drugs most often employed. Drug reactions are common, and the good clinician must be aware of potential toxic side effects and modify therapy accordingly. Supportive treatment for TB is also of great importance. Proper nutrition and the treatment of other co-infections should be emphasized.

Prevention

Whenever possible, respiratory isolation precautions should be taken when treating actively infected individuals. Ideally, these patients should be kept in a separate ward until they have received at least 2 weeks of treatment.

In countries with a high prevalence of TB, BCG vaccine, a live attenuated vaccine derived from M. *bovis*, can be given intradermally. It should be part of the childhood vaccine series. It affords little protection to adults.

Rabies

Rabies is a zoonosis, a disease primarily of wild and domestic animals that is occasionally transmitted to human beings. Another name for it is "hydrophobia": fear of water. The person is thirsty but an attempt to drink brings violent painful muscular contractions, accompanied by extreme fear. The danger of contracting this disease from an infected dog's saliva has been known from ancient times. Rabies virus is the prototype of the genus *lyssavirus* (Greek, from *lyssa*, meaning rage/frenzy) of the large family of Rhabdoviridae. The bullet-shaped rabies virion measures approximately 180 × 75 nm. Rabies is enzootic worldwide except for Australia and a number of islands, such as the British Isles. A frightening annual mortality is still recorded in certain countries.

Rabies most commonly follows the bite of an infected dog that has virus-bearing saliva. However, a dog can bite a cat, who which also can be an agent in the transmission. Other common animal reservoirs include foxes, bats, raccoons, and skunks. Virus-laden saliva is inoculated through the skin, often into muscle. The virus spreads centripetally along axons to the brain. This spread may take months, which, fortunately, gives time for the rabies vaccine to produce levels of neutralizing antibody. However, severe bites, especially if on the head or neck, are associated with short incubation periods. The incubation period is between 20 and 90 days in at least 60% of cases, but it has varied from 4 days to 19 years.

Clinical Features

Approximately one-third of patients experience prodromal symptoms 3 to 7 days before the onset of the disease. These symptoms are usually nonspecific: fever, headache, myalgias, sore throat, irritability, and anxiety. Subsequently, either the symptoms of furious or dumb rabies develop, depending on whether the infection is predominantly in the brain or spinal cord. Usually, rabies transmitted to man by dogs results in furious rabies, while bat transmitted rabies tends to cause dumb rabies.

Furious rabies is characterized by hydrophobia—a combination of spasm of the inspiratory muscle and terror in response to attempts to drink water—or even the sight, sound, or mere mention of drinking water. Other external stimuli, such as bright lights or loud sounds, can excite a similar spasm. The spasms occur in full consciousness, are painful, are associated with a feeling of terror, and can end in convulsions and opisthotonus. The patient may develop hallucinations, delusions, or aggressive behavior, such as spitting or biting. Periods of hallucinations, during which the patient becomes wild and aggressive, alternate with lucid intervals. Other signs include meningism, cardiac arrhythmias, upper-motor neuron lesions, fasciculation, and involuntary movements. Stimulation of the autonomic nervous system can cause lachrymation, hypersalivation, sweating, and fluctuating temperature and blood pressure. Death usually results from cardiac or respiratory arrest. Even in intensive-care facilities, 35% of rabies patients die early during hydrophobic spasms. In most cases, death occurs within 7 days of onset of symptoms. While a few well-documented rabies patients have survived with prolonged, intensive supportive care, in developing countries, it is invariably fatal.

Paralytic or dumb rabies appears to be less common than furious rabies in humans and is mostly associated with bat transmitted infection. Numbness and paralysis develop in the bitten limb, and the paralysis ascends, affecting all muscle control including sphincters, swallowing, and respiration. Usually, death is slower and takes 2 to 3 weeks. Cerebral congestion and a few petechial hemorrhages are usual findings in rabies encephalitis but not gross cerebral edema. In the differential diagnosis, one has to consider the possibility of a psychiatric illness. Bizarre behavior may be a sign of other systemic diseases, such as cerebral malaria or African trypanosomiasis. One must also consider the possibility of tetanus. However, in tetanus, there is constant muscle rigidity, giving the sign of "lockjaw."

Treatment

After being bitten, the management of animal bites is of prime importance. The wound should be scrubbed vigorously with a detergent and rinsed with copious amounts of water. A viricidal agent should be used to swab the wound thoroughly. In an emergency, wound cleansing can be carried out immediately; on admission to a hospital, a thorough washing should be repeated under local anesthesia, or general anesthesia if required. Deep bites should be surgically explored, debrided, and irrigated. Under no account should any bites be sutured or occlusive dressing used. Any wound should be allowed to heal by secondary intention. The agony of a patient with rabies must be relieved by heavy sedation with diazepam along with chlorpromazine if necessary.

Nutrition and fluids can be given intravenously. The patient should be given a tetanus vaccine, if appropriate, and an antimicrobial agent may be used for any potential bacterial infection.

The patient should then be assessed for post-exposure treatment for rabies, using both rabies immune globulin (RIG) as well as a series of vaccine inoculations depending on the patient's pre-exposure vaccination history, and on the nature of the bite or exposure. If the bite consists of a lick of intact skin, scratches, abrasions, without bleeding; or minor bites on covered areas of arms, trunk, or legs; and the animal is available for inspection, then a course of 5 rabies vaccinations should be commenced. If the animal is still alive after 10 days, treatment can be stopped. If the animal is unavailable for inspection, then both rabies hyperimmune serum and vaccine should be given. In the event of a major exposure, such as licks of mucosa or major multiple bites on the face, head, or neck, the patient should receive both serum and a full series of vaccine.

The usual post-exposure regime of rabies cell culture vaccine is a series of five injections: 1.0 ml of vaccine intramuscularly on day 0, 3, 7, 14, and 28. In many developing countries, rabies vaccine is very expensive, and multiple site intradermal regimes can then be used to minimize the actual volume of vaccine needed, thereby optimizing the scarce and expensive resources. Several regimens are approved by WHO. One such regimen, used with success in Thailand, requires 0.1 ml intradermally in eight sites on day 0; four sites are used on day 7, and one site on day 28 and 91. Other reduced dose multiple site regimens are approved and can be found on the WHO website. If the patient has received an adequate pre-exposure regimen of rabies vaccine, then regardless of the nature of the bite, rabies immune globulin (RIG) need not be used, and two further inoculations of vaccine are given on day 0 and day 3. No deaths from rabies have been reported in anyone who has had pre-exposure treatment and post-exposure booster injections.

Prevention

Prevention is provided by pre exposure prophylaxis for anyone residing in an area where there is danger of rabies; it should also be given to those who are visiting endemic areas, even for short periods but who are likely to have significant exposure. Travelers to foreign countries where rabies is endemic should be advised to avoid contact with animals, and what steps to take if bitten. Long-stay travelers, and those going off the beaten track, along with those at occupational risk from contact with rabid animals, may wish to consider pre-exposure prophylactic vaccine. A pre-exposure course consists of 3 doses of tissue culture vaccine given intramuscularly (IM) on days 0, 7, and 21 or 28. An alternative is intradermal injections of 0.1 ml at the same intervals. Chloroquine taken as malaria prophylaxis can suppress the antibody response to intradermal pre-exposure treatment; in such cases, the vaccine must be given intramuscularly (IM).

Rabies hyperimmune serum is also used to prevent rabies in major exposures and also in any patient who may be immunosuppressed for any reason. The serum is given in a dose of 20 units per kg bw; one-half of the volume is injected in and around the wound, and the remainder is given IM at a distant site from where the vaccine is injected. In small children, the amount of serum required may be small, and dilution may be necessary to give a sufficient volume adequately to infiltrate the wound site.

The control of rabies in domestic animals relies on the regular vaccination of domestic pets, and on public campaigns to encourage owners to keep domestic pets away from wild animals. Any domestic animal bitten by a wild animal should be brought to veterinary attention.

Health educational programs should be used to encourage the public to stay away from wild animals and to avoid handling animals that are sick or dying. Any animal behaving strangely should be reported to the relevant authorities. Members of the public who have been in significant contact with a potentially or proven rabid animal should be offered full post-exposure treatment.

Physicians and nurses caring for rabies patients are at high risk. The patient's saliva is potentially infective. Everyone in contact with a rabies patient should be protected by full-barrier nursing techniques, including the use of goggles. Infection through conjunctiva can occur, and, as already noted, rabid patients often spit and bite.

Leprosy

Leprosy has been known since antiquity. The Egyptians noted it among their slaves 1,300 years before Christ. Confucius mentions it, as do the early Vedic physicians of India. The disease is recorded in the Old Testament, and a famous parable in the New Testament describes a well-organized system of community isolation against leprous persons. It is likely that many unrelated dermatologic lesions were considered leprous in biblical times. The disease was apparently very prevalent in Europe during the Middle Ages but did not exist in the Americas before the advent of the white man in the fifteenth century. The incidence in North America was later markedly increased by the importation of infected slaves from areas of Africa where leprosy was endemic.

The cause of leprosy was unknown to the ancients. It was believed to be a punishment of God, and patients with leprosy were ostracized more for religious and aesthetic reasons than as a public health measure. Later, it was thought to be a hereditary disease and, possibly, a venereal one. Linnaeus attributed it to eating fish contaminated with nematodes. In the nineteenth century, Jonathan Hutchinson expounded the fish theory; and in the first edition of Osler's textbook (1898), this possibility is strongly considered. As late as 1908, Balfour wrote in *Recent Advances in Tropical Medicine* that "one notes the tendency to attribute the disease in the first instance to the bites of insects."

The disease is common in the Indian subcontinent, tropical Africa, and South America. The introduction of multidrug therapy regimens has led to a dramatic decline in the prevalence of the disease although a number of new cases are still diagnosed, emphasizing still that transmission continues.

The Organism

In 1873, the Norwegian physician Gerhard Hansen described a bacillus consistently found in the nodules of patients with leprosy, a finding that predated Koch's discovery of the tubercle bacillus by 8 years. *Mycobacterium leprae* is morphologically indistinguishable from the tubercle bacillus, and like that organism, is acid- and alkali-fast. It has a very slow multiplication rate, dividing only once every 14 days, and although highly infective, it has a low virulence. In the human body, the organism grows best where the temperature is below that of the body core. It cannot be grown on culture media, but a limited infection can be induced in footpads of mice. The main source of organisms used in laboratory research is the nine-banded armadillo, which is an animal with a low body temperature and a primitive immunological system.

Pathology

Leprosy is an infection primarily involving the superficial nerves and skin. The immunological state of the infected person determines the type of disease that develops. *M. leprae* is an intracellular bacteria to which the body responds through the cell mediated immune system. When immunity is high, the invading bacilli are engulfed and destroyed without evidence of clinical infection. With a lesser degree of resistance, the organisms provoke a brisk lymphocytic response with aggregations of round, epithelial, and giant cells forming noncaseating granulomas in the corium and nerves. When the cell mediated immune response to this organism is grossly deficient, there is no lymphocytic infiltration, and the macrophages become distended with dividing bacilli, which they are unable to destroy. A brisk humoral antibody response is ineffective, and the bacilli are soon disseminated throughout the body. It is mainly in the superficial tissues and organs that pathological lesions develop.

A measurement of the level of cell-mediated immunity to *M. leprae* is provided by the lepromin test. The antigen is a biologically standardized suspension of killed *M. leprae,* which is injected intradermally into the flexor aspect of the arm. When positive, a granulomatous nodule, develops after 4 weeks, Mitsuda reaction. This reaction is positive in 95% of healthy people and in those with paucibacillary leprosy, but negative in those with multibacillary leprosy. It is, therefore, a prognostic rather than a diagnostic test.

There is still debate as to how infection is acquired, but family contacts of lepromatous patients have 10 times the incidence of leprosy when compared with the general population. In lepromatous patients, the lepra bacilli are found in large numbers in sweat glands, sebaceous glands, and hair follicles, but few are excreted through the intact skin. On the other hand, several million organisms may be discharged each day in the nasal secretions, and these may remain viable for 8 to 10 days. It thus seems possible that infection is acquired via the upper respiratory tract in a manner rather similar to tuberculosis.

There are many different systems of classifying clinical leprosy; we list in decreasing order of immune response as follows:

1. Tuberculoid leprosy (TL)
2. Borderline leprosy
   a. Borderline tuberculoid leprosy (BT)
   b. Borderline borderline leprosy (BB)
   c. Borderline lepromatous leprosy (BL)
3. Lepromatous leprosy (LL)

TL and BT are also termed "paucibacillary leprosy," and BB, BL, and LL as "multibacillary leprosy."

Clinical Features

The incubation period is usually prolonged, and although leprosy has been detected in infants as young as 4 months of age, most infections acquired in childhood first present between the ages of 20 to 35 years. In a group of American servicemen infected in the tropics, the incubation period for tuberculoid leprosy averaged 4 years, and 10 years for lepromatous leprosy. Leprosy may develop rapidly, but in the great majority, the disease starts with one or more inconspicuous, hypopigmented, or erythematous areas of the skin. Over months or years, these may either disappear completely or develop into one of the recognizable types of leprosy. This early stage is termed *indeterminate leprosy*.

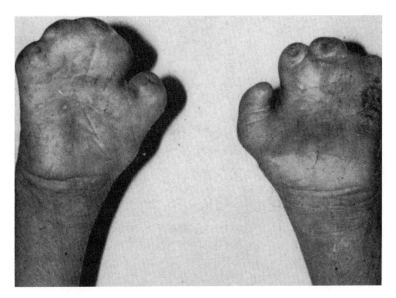

FIGURE 15: Loss of fingers and toes, due to nerve and vascular damage as well as trauma, occurs in tuberculoid and borderline leprosy.

In *tuberculoid leprosy*, the lesions are either single, or if more than one, asymmetrical. Common sites are the face, lateral aspects of the limbs, buttocks, and scapulae. They appear as annular plaques or macules with sharp, raised, clear-cut, erythematous edges that slope gently to a flattened hypopigmented center. The surface is rough and dry, and typically, there is loss of all forms of sensation. The lesion expands slowly at the periphery, with subsequent healing and repigmentation starting at the center.

Enlarged tender nerve fibrils may be felt under the skin around the lesion. Another classical feature in this form of leprosy is the gradual thickening of nerves, particularly the ulna at the elbow, the radial and median at the wrist, the lateral popliteal as it winds round the head of the fibula, and the posterior auricular nerve in the neck. This nerve thickening is associated with loss of related function.

The lesions of *borderline leprosy* are much more varied. Multiple asymmetrical macules, plaques, and annular or bizarre-shaped bands appear in crops. In contrast with *tuberculoid leprosy*, the lesions tend to be dome shaped with an elevated center. A common form appears as succulent rings surrounding healthy skin with one side forming a sharp margin, the other side gradually merging into healthy skin. Loss of sensation over the lesions is not marked, but involvement of the main nerve trunks is early and widespread. Indeed, some patients present with nerve palsies without any obvious skin involvement (neural leprosy). Involvement of the fifth and seventh cranial nerves may lead to lagophthalmos and exposure keratitis; other patients develop clawhand or footdrop. This is an unstable form of leprosy and may evolve toward either the tuberculoid or lepromatous forms.

Lepromatous leprosy is a malignant and very stable form of disease. It starts as a rash composed of numerous, small, vague, hypopigmented macules scattered symmetrically over the face, trunk, and limbs. In dark skins, the macules may have a coppery hue, while in white skins, they are erythematous. The affected skin may appear shiny or greasy but is not anesthetic. As time goes on, the skin becomes increasingly thickened and infiltrated. At a later stage, papules and nodules may appear.

When the face is affected, the thickening of the skin can occur so gradually that it may pass unnoticed, but lateral thinning of the eyebrows and thickening of the ear lobes are useful confirmatory signs. Eventually, these gross changes produce a so-called "leonine facies." The peripheral nerves undergo slow but steady symmetrical thickening, followed by increasing loss of peripheral sensation and a "glove and stocking" type of anesthesia.

The nasal mucosa may be affected causing rhinorrhea, bloodstained discharge and obstruction. Laryngeal involvement results in hoarseness, stridor, and occasionally edema of the glottis. The bacilli also lodge in the ciliary body of the eye, and episcleritis, scleritis, and keratitis may develop. A devastating iridocyclitis, usually occurring during an episode of erythema nodosum leprosum, is one of the more common causes of blindness in the tropics. Invasion of the testes leads to acute orchitis, impotency, sterility, and gynecomastia. Leprous dactylitis and renal failure from glomerular nephritis or amyloidosis are other common manifestations of this malignant infection.

Diagnosis

The diagnosis of fully developed leprosy seldom presents difficulty, but by then, the disease will have been present for some years. On the

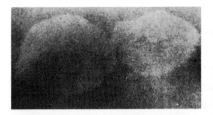

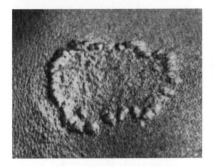

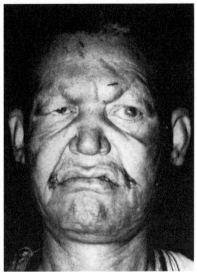

FIGURE 16: *Tuberculoid leprosy*, often misdiagnosed as vitiligo and ringworm. (Top) The maculoanesthetic lesion is flat, discrete, hypopigmented, and insensitive. They may progress to an infiltrated area with raised borders (Bottom). Scrapings from these lesions for *M. leprae* frequently show negative findings, but biopsy will be characteristic.

FIGURE 17: Typical leonine facies of advanced *lepromatous leprosy*. The nodules are concentrated on ears, chin, and malar and interciliary areas. Eyebrow alopecia is marked. Palpebral palsy and corneal lepromata are apparent.

other hand, the vague macules of early lepromatous leprosy are easily missed or difficult to distinguish from tinea versicolor or secondary syphilis. Pure neural forms are often misdiagnosed even in regions where leprosy is common. Leprosy should be suspected in any person who has spent time in the tropics and who has developed a persisting, painless, nonirritating skin lesion or a nerve palsy.

Confirmation of the diagnosis, and classification of the type of leprosy, is achieved by correlating the clinical, bacteriological, and histological findings with the result of a lepromin test. In tuberculoid leprosy, skin smears and nasal scrapings will be negative for acid fast bacilli; a biopsy will reveal noncaseating granulomas bordering the epidermis; the lepromin test will be strongly positive. In patients with lepromatous leprosy, on the other hand, skin smears and nasal scrapings will reveal plentiful *M. leprae*; the biopsy will contain loose granulomas composed of macrophages distended with acid-fast organisms, but the immediate subepidermal zone will be spared; the lepromin test will be negative. The findings in borderline leprosy will be less definite, BT tending to resemble the tuberculoid polar type, and BB and BL the lepromatous type. Confirmation of pure neural leprosy is based on a biopsy taken from a thickened sensory nerve branch. In view of the traditional (if quite irrational) horror and stigma still attached to this disease in many countries, a false-positive diagnosis must be avoided at all costs.

Treatment

The treatment of leprosy has been revolutionized. Patients no longer require segregation and separation from their families and work. They can be treated as outpatients in general purpose clinics, mixing freely with other patients and can be offered the prospect of a complete cure within 6 months to 2 years.

The following clinical classification for treatment control programs has been formulated by WHO:

> Paucibacillary (PB) single lesion leprosy (one skin lesion): A single dose of Rifampicin 600 mg + Ofloxacin 400 mg + Minocycline 100 mg
>
> Paucibacillary (PB) 2 to 5 skin lesions leprosy: Self-administration of 100 mg Dapsone daily + 600 mg Rifampicin monthly for 6 months
>
> Multibacillary (MB) leprosy more than five skin lesions or smear-positive patients: self-administration of 100 mg Dapsone daily + 50 mg Clofazimine daily for 12 months as well as supervised administration of rifampicin 600 mg + clofazimine 300 mg monthly for 12 months

Unfortunately, even effective treatment is often attended by reactions, which can be very damaging unless urgently treated in hospital. Erythema nodosum leprosum (ENL) occurs during treatment in about one-half of patients with multibacillary leprosy. It follows the death of organisms that nevertheless remain *in situ* and antigenically active. Immune complexes are laid down in the blood vessels of the dermis, with activation of complement leading to inflammation. Crops of small, hot, tender nodules erupt on the arms, thighs, and face, and are accompanied by fever, malaise, a leukocytosis, and a raised erythrocyte sedimentation rate (ESR). Immune complex deposition may also occur at other sites, causing swelling or even suppuration in lymph nodes, polyneuritis, dactylitis, and arthritis. Most leprosy-induced episodes of glomerular nephritis with renal failure are due to this reaction. Secondary amyloidosis, another common complication, appears to be closely related to the severity and frequency of these episodes. As mentioned previously, severe iridocyclitis occurs in ENL and frequently results in blindness. Treatment includes strict bed rest, analgesics, thalidomide (except in pregnant women), and an increase in the dose of clofazimine. Prednisolone may also be required in severe reactions. Contrary to previous advice, chemotherapy should be continued throughout the attack.

Other complications related to therapy are "upgrading" and "downgrading" reactions. The former occurs in borderline leprosy when there is improvement in cell mediated immunity. Although there are no constitutional disturbances, acute inflammation of skin and nerves can produce a palsy requiring prednisolone therapy or even surgical decompression. Downgrading reactions, also seen mainly in borderline patients, reflect a worsening of the disease due to ineffective treatment.

Prevention

Preventive measures are directed toward the reduction of the reservoir of infection by providing facilities for diagnosis, treatment, and the surveillance of contacts even in remote rural areas. It is already evident that education and the introduction of less-harsh regimens for treatment have been effective in unmasking many actively infective individuals. Efforts are also being made to increase the resistance of individuals in endemic areas. BCG, although ineffective in Asia, has been shown to give significant protection against leprosy in Africa. Combining BCG and killed *M. leprae* showed no advantage over BCG alone in Malawi and Venezuela. Efforts are being made to produce new vaccines by genetic engineering. Since the introduction of multidrug therapy, the number of cases has fallen dramatically. Within the next few years, it is hoped that newly acquired infections will become rarer and that the elimination of the disease as a public health problem remains a possibility.

Treponemal and Fungal Infections

Tropical Treponematoses

It is thought that treponemal infections evolved in the primeval, moist jungles of Africa, altered in highlands and arid desert communities, and finally halted in an arrested state in the Americas. Between the florid sores of yaws and the limited depigmentation of pinta lie a variety of lesions with a multitude of local names, including *bejel, sita, njovera, dichuchwa,* and *radesyga.* These diseases are of interest because of their endemicity, chronicity, and curability as well as for the light they cast on the more widely diagnosed treponemal disease, venereal syphilis. All treponemal infections are morphologically and serologically indistinguishable; none of the tropical variants are venereal diseases. Some authorities contend that all treponematoses are different manifestations of one disease; nevertheless, clinical and epidemiologic patterns permit the differentiation of yaws from *bejel* and other intermediate forms and from pinta.

Yaws

In common with all tropical treponematoses, yaws is a disease of squalor. It is found in the hot, humid lowlands of Africa, Asia, and Central America, especially where nakedness and crowded conditions are common, and water is scarce. By conservative estimates, more than 50 million persons were infected with yaws before a WHO global therapy program began. As health systems—particularly, surveillance and early therapy programs—have collapsed in parts of war-torn Africa, yaws has reemerged. Although the causative organism, *Treponema pertenue,* is indistinguishable from *T. pallidum,* the natural history of the disease is markedly different from that of syphilis.

Transmission is nonvenereal, with direct contact as the major method of spread, and mechanical conveyance by the *Hippelates pallipes* fly as a minor means. The primary lesion is an inconspicuous papule that is found most frequently in children of from 2 to 5 years of age. The "mother" papule, which erupts 3 to 5 weeks after infection, is pruritic but painless, and it may enlarge into a hypertrophic papilloma of 2 cm. Papillomata often erupt over the body surface within a few weeks after the initial lesion, but they may not appear for years. The concept of latency is particularly important to the understanding of the course of yaws, for "early" lesions can erupt long after the initial sore, and several crops of early lesions may appear within the first 5 years of infection, each healing without evidence of scarring.

Secondary skin sores are more numerous and disfiguring. These "daughter" or "typical" yaws lesions are yellow, raised, wart- or raspberry-like, and often have central ulcerations. Serpiginous and circinate papillomata, mucosal plaques, and hyperkeratotic or ulcerating lesions of the palms and the soles are other varieties of early yaws. Once again,

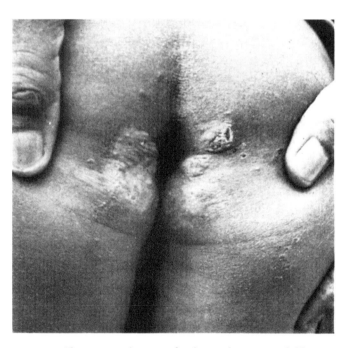

FIGURE 18: Characteristic location of early yaws lesions in a child.

long latent periods may separate multiple secondary relapses, and healing is without scar formation.

Bone and joint lesions of early yaws also heal spontaneously without residual damage. Polydactylitis is characteristic of early yaws in children. Periostitis is frequent, especially involving the radius, ulna, and nasal maxilla; ganglions and transient hydroarthrosis may occur. The etiological relationship of yaws to sabre tibia has not been proved.

Within 5 years of infection, yaws can become a destructive disease, and "late" lesions of both skin and bones produce permanent damage. Internal organs are not involved. Gummatous nodules with central ulceration may persist as indolent sores or resolve with residual scar and keloid formation. Marked hyperkeratosis of the palms and the soles may cause Dupuytren-like contractures. Gummatous periostitis and osteitis produce an x-ray of mixed translucency and density. Osteomyelitis, suppurative dactylitis, and complete collapse of the nasal septum (gangosa) may complicate the course of late yaws.

The diagnosis of yaws can be confirmed by visualization of *T. pertenue* in dark field preparations or on stained smears obtained from ulcer edges. Immunological evidence provided by positive treponemal infections cannot be differentiated in the serology laboratory. Partial cross immunity appears to exist with syphilis; when yaws is eradicated, the incidence of venereal syphilis rises. Nonetheless, there have been many cases in which double infection with *T. pallidum* and *T. pertenue* has been demonstrated.

Penicillin cures yaws. Almost all early infections are healed after a course of 500,000 units daily for 7 days. Late cases usually respond to a regimen of 1 million units daily for 10 days. In mass programs, a single injection of 1.2 million units of long-acting penicillin has proved effective.

Intermediate Forms

Yaws becomes less florid as the geography changes from moist lowland to dry savannah. Along the desert borders of Africa and the Middle East, *bejel* and other endemic syphilides are the dominant nonvenereal treponemal infections. The onset of these diseases usually occurs later in childhood than does that of yaws. Lesions are concentrated on moist areas such as the mouth, axilla, inguinal area, and rectum. The frequency of sores on the buccal mucosal junctions caused the common drinking cup to be incriminated as a mechanical means of spread. Late palmar lesions and bone destruction are common, but no organ damage occurs. Serological tests for syphilis are positive, and although visualization of treponema from wound aspirates is desirable, there is nothing pathognomonic in their morphology. Treatment with penicillin is curative.

Pinta

Throughout much of tropical America, another nonvenereal treponemal infection exists. Pinta (thus called from the Spanish word for "spot") is a purely cutaneous disease caused by *T. carateum*. Primary lesions, observed only under experimental conditions, appear 10 to 16 days after artificial inoculation. The natural means of transmission is uncertain; direct contact is presumed to be the major method of spread although vector transmission by both *Simulium* and *Hippelates* flies has been proved to be possible. The secondary lesions, or pintids, are scaly, squamous papules on an erythematous base. As the lesions become inactive, achromia becomes more prominent. These areas of slaty depigmentation are usually bilateral and symmetric and are associated with concurrent desquamation, lichenization, and hyperkeratosis. There is no latent period in pinta, and the tertiary lesions evolve from pintids. Treponemas can be found in juice expressed from scrapings of pintids, but they are rare in the achromic, late lesions. Penicillin will cure pinta but will not reverse late depigmentary changes.

Fungal Infections

Fungi occur as ubiquitous saprophytes of the soil in most tropical regions. Fortunately, they are mostly pathogens of low invasiveness, and serious systemic disease occurs primarily when cell-mediated immunity is compromised. Cryptococcal meningoencephalitis, histoplasmosis, and candidiasis are important opportunistic infections of AIDS in the tropics. Far more common, however, and the cause of

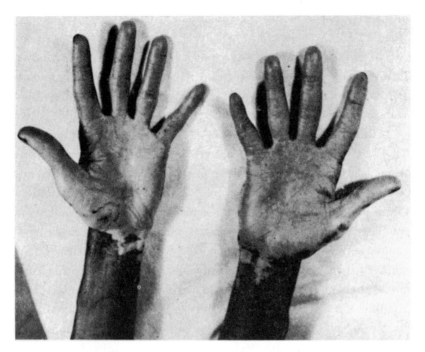

FIGURE 19: Classical late pinta, showing total achromia of the palms with moderate hyperkeratosis.

much human suffering, are other superficial and systemic fungal diseases.

Cutaneous fungal infection

Skin infection with *Malassezia furfur* and *M. tropica* is almost universal in many tropical countries. Only the most superficial layer of the skin is affected. In dark skins, the infected areas are hypopigmented with a characteristic fluffy appearance, as if covered with fine dust. The areas most commonly affected are between the scapulae and the front of the chest. The fungi often cannot be cultured, but the mycelia and spores may be demonstrated in skin scrapings.

Rhinosporidiosis is a chronic granulomatous condition due to R. *seeberi* affecting mainly the nasal mucosa. It is endemic in India, Sri Lanka, east Africa, and parts of Latin America. Pedunculated lesions of the anterior nares cause obstruction with epistaxis. The lesions are highly vascular, friable, polypoid growths with a granular surface; they are pink/red in color and bleed when touched. The optimal therapy is complete excision; otherwise, recurrence is the rule. Histological examination of the excised lesion reveals sharply defined globular cysts filled with round, darkly staining spores.

Three related species of black molds, of which the most important are *Chadopsoria*, cause the condition known as *dermatitis verrucosa* or *mossy foot*, seen mainly in South America. The fungus is inoculated into a wound, nearly always on the foot. A small, warty plaque follows, which gradually extends. Satellite lesions appear and eventually grow into large verrucose tumor–like masses, often pedunculated, like small cauliflowers. They are friable, hemorrhage easily, and produce a foul-smelling discharge. Diffuse hyperkeratosis follows, and secondary infection is common. The lesions are painless, but over years, extend slowly. Examination of the crust or a biopsy will reveal thick-walled, dark brown bodies that multiply by fission rather than by budding. In the early stages, excision with electrocautery may be curative, but later, the only remedy available may be amputation.

Subcutaneous fungal infections

Madura foot is endemic in arid lands stretching in a band from India across northern Sudan to Senegal. It accounts for a definable percentage of hospital admissions in Khartoum. The infecting organisms are eumycetes, true fungi of which the best known is *Madurella mycetoma*; certain aerobic actinomycetes, and hyphal producing bacteria, such as *Streptomyces* and *Nocardia* species, are among the other etiologic agents. These organisms abound in dry, sandy soil and usually enter bare feet on the contaminated thorns of acacia trees. Once introduced, the organisms grow and reproduce eliciting a granulomatous reaction along fascial planes with necrosis and multiple abscess formation. Adjacent bones are then involved, and the foot becomes intersected by sinuses and fistulae that ultimately erupt on to the skin, discharging mucopurulent material containing multicolored grains: black or dark brown with *M. mycetoma*, yellow or red with *Streptomyces*.

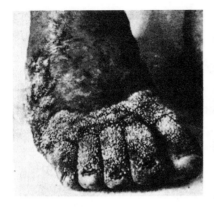

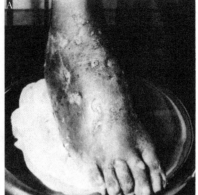

FIGURE 20: (Above)
Mossy foot in a Brazilian patient.

FIGURE 21:
(A) A Madura foot in a Sudanese patient.
(B) The original camera lucida drawing
of a mycetoma.

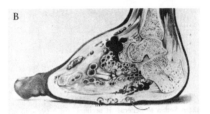

The earliest lesions are hard, painless nodules in the subcutaneous tissue. They gradually enlarge and form extensive abscesses that transform the foot into a tumor, the surface of which is studded with fresh nodules, discharging sinuses, and scars. The lack of pain and constitutional symptoms accounts for the fact that patients often seek care with grossly advanced lesions. The foot is affected in 75% to 80% of cases, but leg, hand, buttock, and skull may also be involved. In young patients, a mycetoma can present as a painless bony swelling at the upper end of the tibia or lower end of the ulna; x-rays demonstrate a cystic matrix.

A fully developed mycetoma is not a difficult diagnostic challenge, whereas the early small nodule under the healthy skin is less distinctive. In both cases, it is essential, from a therapeutic point of view, to identify the infecting organism. The color of the grains, if present, helps. Confirmation is obtained by culture, histopathology, and precipitation tests. Actinomycete infections may respond to long-term treatment with ketoconazole or septrin, dapsone, streptomycin, and rifampicin; eumycete infections have been amenable only to surgery, sometimes involving amputation.

Deep fungal infections

Other fungal infections are acquired by inhalation of spores as well as by subcutaneous inoculation and, in both circumstances, may produce localized as well as disseminated disease.

Histoplasma capsulatum, a dimorphic fungus, is a widely distributed soil saprophyte in south and east Africa, southeast Asia, northern Australia, and Latin America. The fungus flourishes in soil contaminated by bat or bird droppings, and human infection usually occurs through inhalation of asexual spores. Most infections remain subclinical and are recognized only as pulmonary calcifications on routine chest x-rays, but a particularly heavy infection may present as an acute pulmonary illness.

After an incubation period of 2 weeks, there is an acute onset of headache, fatigue, malaise, myalgias, a "brassy" cough, dyspnea on exertion, and sometimes pleuritic pain. There may be rigors and a fever rising to 105F. Although clinical examination of the chest may be normal, the x-ray reveals diffuse shadowing, with or without enlargement of the hilar lymph nodes. The white cell count and the erythrocyte sedimentation rate (ESR) remain normal. The illness usually clears spontaneously within 6 weeks, but pulmonary histoplasmosis in older individuals may result in a chronic, bilateral fibrocaseous, cavitating disease, closely resembling pulmonary tuberculosis.

Disseminated *H. capsulatum* infection may present as an illness closely resembling kala azar. Confusion between these two conditions is further heightened as both etiologic organisms are found as 1 to 5 micron, rounded bodies within macrophages. A peculiar form of histoplasmosis is endemic in the Malayan peninsula. It starts with painful ulceration in the mouth, pharynx, larynx, or around the anus; if untreated, generalized dissemination follows. This is often associated with acute adrenal cortical failure. The majority of cases described have been in Europeans with incubation periods up to 30 years.

In west and central Africa, *Histoplasma duboisii* is endemic. In the filamentous form, the fungus is identical to *H. capsulatum*, but in the yeast form in the human body, it is four to five times as large, measuring up to 20 micron in diameter. Patients may present with flat papules, which develop into dome-shaped, sessile nodules with central ulcers and rolled edges. As they enlarge, the center heals, producing annular lesions, which although painless, can persist for years. Some patients develop localized cold abscesses in bones with sinuses discharging on to the skin; common sites are the skull (including the orbit), ribs, scapula, and sternum.

The diagnosis of histoplasmosis is confirmed by growing the fungus on Sabouraud's medium and by recognizing the yeast-like forms in discharges or biopsy material. Special stains such as hexamine (methenamine) silver or periodic acid Schiff are required. Early histoplasmosis often clears spontaneously and requires no treatment. More persistent infections may respond to ketoconazole; disseminated infection demands treatment with amphotericin B supplemented by flucytosine. Amphotericin should be administered in a 5% dextrose solution, using scalp vein needles in distal veins and changing the site of each infusion. While toxic side effects are common, and some degree of renal damage is almost inevitable, it offers the only hope of cure.

Paracoccidioidomycosis or *South American blastomycosis* is the most widespread systemic mycosis of Latin America. *Paracoccidioides braziliensis* infection is thought to be acquired by cleaning teeth with fragments of contaminated wood and by chewing various plant stems. The primary lesion is nearly always in the mouth and consists of erythematous, ulcerated areas with tiny yellow and red spots, giving a mulberry-like appearance. The lesions spread to the face as verrucous or papillomatous, heavily encrusted vegetations. Draining abscesses develop in the cervical and submaxillary lymph nodes, and eventually, multiple pustular or ulcerative lesions may spread over the body. Occasionally, the lesions may be confined to the gastrointestinal tract or lungs. Diffuse dissemination may occur, as in generalized histoplasmosis. This infection responds to long-term therapy with ketoconazole, but intravenous amphotericin B may be required. Relapses are common.

A dimorphic fungus, *Blastomycoses dermatitidis*, causing *North American blastomycosis*, is also endemic in east and South Africa. The source of infection is unknown. Human disease is caused by inoculation of spores beneath the skin producing a local lesion, or following inhalation, a pulmonary involvement. Cutaneous granulomatous tumors contain actively budding yeast-like cells. Single or multiple elevated lesions, studded with tiny pustules, develop on the face, arms, legs, and trunk. There may be raised erythematous, sharply demarcated patches, which can be mistaken for tuberculoid leprosy. Pulmonary symptoms include cough, blood stained sputum, anorexia, wasting, and fever. Generalized dissemination may lead to abscess formation in the liver, spleen, bone, kidneys, and not infrequently, in the brain. The yeasts are approximately the same size as those of *H. duboisii* but are distinguished by having multiple nuclei. Once again, early infection may be suppressed by ketoconazole, but amphotericin B is required for a cure of disseminated disease.

Diarrheal Diseases

Cholera

Cholera has existed in the Ganges Delta since time immemorial, but in the nineteenth century, six great pandemics spread as far and rapidly as man was then able to travel. A seventh pandemic due to the El Tor biotype began in Indonesia in 1961, spreading throughout southern Asia and into Africa, killing tens of thousands. In Bangladesh and India, the classical vibrio biotype appears to be regaining its dominant position, and outbreaks continue to occur early each winter and spring, accounting for 6% of fatal cases of childhood diarrhea in the area. Cholera is also a threat in many humanitarian emergencies; following conflict and natural disasters, people are often forced to live together in refugee enclaves with inadequate clear water supplies and grossly unsanitary conditions. An outbreak in Haiti in 2010 that killed thousands of refugees is a reminder of the virulence of this infection.

The Organism

Vibrio cholerae is a motile, gram-negative bacillus shaped like a comma, with a single polar flagellum. It is distinguished from other morphologically identical vibrios by agglutination with group OI type serum. There are two biotypes: the classical and El Tor; and three serotypes: Inaba, Ogawa, and Hikojima. These vibrios flourish in the alkaline, bile-enriched environment of the small intestine; a common laboratory medium for cholera isolation is the alkaline agar (TCBS) medium. In positive cultures, round, yellow, smooth colonies appear after 18 hours. In 1992, a new strain of *V. cholerae*, 0139 Bengal, appeared in India and caused an epidemic in a population that was largely immune to cholera caused by *V. cholerae* OI strains. Outbreaks have since occurred in other areas of south Asia.

Transmission is from human to human via the anal-oral route and most frequently follows the ingestion of water or food contaminated with cholera stools. Because the bacterium is readily destroyed in the stomach acid, ingestion of large quantities of water favors infection, and hypochlorhydric or achlorhydric individuals are particularly vulnerable.

Pathology

The vibrios adhere to the brush border membrane of the small intestinal mucosa where they secrete choleragen, a toxin that is composed of two subunits. The B subunit binds to a specific receptor, while the A subunit penetrates the brush border where, after cleavage, it activates adenylate cyclase, resulting in the conversion of adenosine triphosphate to cyclic adenosine monophosphate. This enzyme promotes increased chloride, sodium, and water secretion into the intestinal lumen while inhibiting the reabsorptive mechanism.

In the small intestinal lumen, there is a massive accumulation of fluid containing sodium and chloride in concentrations roughly similar to that in the plasma. However, the concentrations of potassium and bicarbonate roughly double. This results in dehydration, isonatremic acidosis, and hemoconcentration. The potassium loss is masked by the movement of potassium out of the cells into the plasma. It is this internal loss of fluid and electrolyte imbalance that leads to rapid death from hypovolemic shock, acidosis, and renal failure.

It is interesting that as early as 1831, O'Shaughnessy wrote

> . . . in cholera the blood has lost a large proportion of its water and a great proportion of its natural saline ingredients. Of the free alkali contained in healthy serum, not a particle is present in some cholera patients and barely a trace in others. Urea exists where suppression of urine is a marked symptom.

Until the 1950s, when intestinal biopsy was introduced, it was accepted that in cholera, the small intestinal mucosa was denuded. Now we know that it is morphologically normal; the damage is biochemical and not structural.

Clinical Features

The majority of individuals infected with V. *cholerae* remain asymptomatic or have signs and symptoms of a mild enteritis. In infections with the classical biotype, it is estimated that 14% will develop clinical cholera, while the corresponding figure for the El Tor biotype is only 2%. The period of carriage in asymptomatic persons is about 10 days, but chronic carriers (e.g., "Cholera Dolores") do occur (for more than 3 years), specifically with the El Tor biotype. The small percentage that develop severe cholera, however, presents a clinical picture that is unforgettable.

The incubation period can vary from a few hours to a week, but is most commonly about 48 hours. The onset is usually sudden with an explosive, copious diarrhea in a previously healthy person. The motions, at first fecal and bile-stained, rapidly assume the typical "rice water" appearance, the opalescence being due to mucus content. Diarrhea is effortless and painless, and the volume of fluid passed is almost incredible. It may exceed 1 liter per hour and as much as 20 liters a day so, as one observer noted, ". . . it is unbelievable that the body has sufficient fluid to supply it."

The diarrhea is uncontrolled, and the patient may hardly be aware that it is happening. Vomiting may be copious, but it is unassociated with nausea or retching. A brief rise in temperature may be noted in some patients, but fever is not a significant feature, nor is abdominal pain. Severe muscle cramps, especially affecting the calves of the legs, can become generalized.

Very soon, the effects of dehydration become obvious. Severe thirst develops; the tongue and mouth are dry, the skin loses its turgor, the eyes become sunken, the cheeks collapsed, the lips cyanosed, and the fingers wrinkled (washerwoman's fingers). There may be dyspnea and the breath smells "acidotic." Profound shock is accompanied by coldness of the extremities with a rapid, low-volume, or sometimes impalpable, pulse. The blood pressure is frequently unrecordable. Unless fluid loss is corrected oliguria, anuria, and acute renal failure develop. At first, the patient is restless, but gradually there is an increasing lethargy with a feeble, high-pitched voice. The mind remains clear although terminal stupor or coma may eventually supervene.

Diagnosis

The "rice water" stools are teeming with vibrios, and their characteristic movements may be seen in hanging drop preparations on dark field examination. Their rapid movement is immediately brought to a halt by the addition of a drop of Group Ol polyvalent antiserum. Cultures may be obtained from fresh stool fluid, rectal swabs, or filter paper impregnated with potassium tellurite that has been soaked in liquid stool. Colonies will develop on MacConkey's medium, but not on *Shigella-Salmonella* agar. The vibrios grow best on selective media, such as thiosulphate citrate bile salt sucrose (TCBS) or taurochlolate tellurite gelatin agar. The vibrios are further identified by slide agglutination against Ol antiserum and then against anti Inaba and anti Okawa sera. The biotypes are distinguished by hemolysis of red cells, sensitivity to Group IV phage and polymyxin, and resistance to El Tor Group 5 phage.

Treatment

Rapid intravenous (IV) replacement of fluid and electrolytes is the most important part of the treatment of severe cholera. Like the common cold, cholera cures itself, provided that dehydration can be rapidly and adequately corrected. Patients recover with amazing rapidity, and an apparently moribund patient may, after a few hours, be sitting up and asking for food or drink.

The volume of fluid lost should be replaced within 4 hours. A large bore needle is passed into an anticubital vein, and the infusion is delivered at a rate of 500 to 1,000 ml per hour until a strong radial pulse can be felt. The drip is then continued more slowly until adequate rehydration, as judged by the patient's clinical condition, has been achieved. Evidence for this is provided by the cessation of vomiting and cramps, as well as restoration of pulse volume, blood pressure, skin tone, and a normal urinary output. Several infusion fluids are used for this purpose, the ideal for adults being normal saline and 1/6 molar lactate in a ratio of 2:1; if this is not available, normal saline alone is usually quite satisfactory. Tetracycline should be given in a dose of 40 mg per kg bw daily (maximum 4 g daily) in 4 divided doses for 2 days.

Following initial rehydration, the patient may continue to have severe diarrhea for several days, and this fluid with its electrolytes must be replaced. The amount lost may be conveniently measured by nursing the patient on a "cholera cot," which is a stretcher with a hole in the center so that the liquid excreta can be collected—and measured—in containers beneath the bed. At this stage, fluid can be administered orally, and a suitable low-osmolality glucose-salt solution can be given. Rice powder instead of glucose can be used. A number of prepackaged commercial preparations are available. Tetracycline, doxycycline, and furazolidone reduce the volume and duration of diarrhea. A single dose of doxycycline 300 mg is the most convenient.

Prevention

The importance of adequate sanitation and hygiene was highlighted when the last pandemic reached the shores of the Mediterranean, where only very limited outbreaks occurred. In Africa, public health attention to wells and other sources of drinking water gave more protection than vaccination. Prophylactic tetracycline proved not only ineffective, but its use in east Africa led to the development of resistant organisms. The vaccine now in general use is also unsatisfactory, giving only partial protection for a short time. New vaccines are being developed, one promising one being an orally administered B subunit killed-whole-cell vaccine (RBS-WC) containing the B subunit of cholera toxin with killed whole cells of both biotypes and Inaba and Ogawa serotypes. It has been shown to be both safe and protective even in HIV-infected patients. New vaccines are now available in Europe but are not yet approved by the FDA for use in the United States.

Shigellosis

Bacillary dysentery due to infection with *Shigella* remains one of the most important tropical diseases. Recent years have seen large epidemics of severe dysentery in South America, central Africa, and Bangladesh, in which the case mortality rate has been higher than in cholera.

The Organism

Shigella are gram-negative, noncapsulated, nonsporing, nonmotile, nonlactose-fermenting rods. On the basis of fermentation reactions and serology, they are divided into four groups, each group containing several serotypes. These groups are *S. dysenteriae*, *S. flexneri*, *S. boydii*, and *S. sonnei*. In the tropics, *S. flexneri* is most prevalent, while *S. dysenteriae* type 1 has been responsible for most of the epidemics of severe dysentery.

Pathology

This is the most communicable of all bacterial enteric infections as very few organisms are required to initiate disease. The organisms multiply in the colon where, as with cholera, they attach to the mucosa, allowing subunits to enter the epithelial cells. Unlike cholera, however, shigellae produce acute inflammation, necrosis, epithelial ulceration, and hemorrhage. The whole mucosa becomes hyperemic, edematous, and friable, and bleeds easily. Later, superficial serpiginous ulcers may develop, and in extreme cases, progress to gangrene and mucosal sloughing. Microscopically, there is vascular engorgement, intense infiltration with plasma cells, and necrosis starting around the crypts.

Clinical Features

The incubation period varies but is usually about 5 days. Mildly affected patients have a short 2 to 3 day illness, passing six to eight loose stools daily with or without a small amount of blood and mucus. By contrast, the severe illness starts with an abrupt onset of fever, malaise, headache, anorexia, and often severe abdominal colic. At first, the motions are fairly normal, but soon give place to brown, watery stools with flecks of blood-stained mucus, and finally just bloody mucus, the patient passing 20 to 60 stools daily consisting of small quantities of gelatinous, blood-stained mucus that stick to the bed pan.

According to the amount of blood present, the stools have been described as "pink frog spawn" or "red currant jelly." Such motions contain almost no fecal material and are odorless. Colic continues to be severe, and tenesmus is a distressing symptom, occurring in spasms lasting for one-half hour after defecation, sometimes accompanied by dysuria. Vomiting may occur at the onset, but it is not a prominent symptom. Fever may continue for several days and is usually higher at night. Seizures are a frequent complication in children.

On physical examination, the tongue is furred, the abdomen flat or scaphoid, and there is tenderness over the descending colon. The degree of this tenderness and its extent is a guide to the severity of the attack. Untreated, the illness lasts 2 to 3 weeks before the diarrhea begins to abate and the motions progress from liquid, fecal stools to semiformed pultaceous ones, and finally to a normal, formed evacuation. Blood is the first constituent to disappear.

Diagnosis

The diagnosis in severely affected patients is usually clear from the clinical features; in those mildly affected, it is suggested by the presence of blood and pus cells in stool smears. Confirmation is obtained by the inoculation of a stool specimen or rectal swab on MacConkey's agar, followed by subculturing nonlactose fermenting colonies on *Salmonella-Shigella* agar. The organisms are further characterized by conventional biochemical procedures and slide agglutination.

Treatment

Dehydration, if present, requires treatment with oral rehydration solution, but narcotic-related drugs to control the frequency of diarrhea should generally be avoided. Unfortunately, these organisms, especially *S. dysenteriae* type 1, have become increasingly resistant to antibacterial drugs. Ampicillin and cotrimoxazole are still widely used. In many countries, the only effective drugs available are nalidixicid acid, the fluoroquinolones, or azithromycin. Vitamin A reduces the severity of shigellosis in children in areas where this dietary deficiency is common.

Prevention

Human feces are the only source of shigellosis, and in this regard, the mildly affected person and the convalescent carriers are of particular importance. During an outbreak, the carrier rate may reach 10% although it seldom lasts more than 3 to 4 months. Contaminated insects are a particularly significant means of spread; both safe disposal of feces and control of fly populations are important preventative measures. This is particularly critical during the chaos of wartime. Shiga, a Japanese physician, stated that bacillary dysentery was the constant companion of battle and was more fatal to the soldiers than powder and shot.

Diarrhea in Children

Acute gastroenteritis affecting infants and young children is one of the principal causes of mortality in the tropics. Millions of children die each year merely from dehydration complicating diarrhea. The cause lies in the unsanitary conditions in which they have to struggle to survive. In many regions, there is no protected water supply and no adequate waste or sewage facilities. During the first 4 to 6 months of life, children on the breast remain well, but attacks of diarrhea soon commence after the introduction of supplementary feeding. These "feeds" take the form of thin gruels made with water often obtained from contaminated wells, streams, or water holes. The water is seldom boiled, and the gruels are often prepared in the morning and then stand at a temperature of 80°F to 90°F. throughout the day. It is difficult to conceive of a better medium for the growth of many pathogens.

The Organisms

The most significant etiologic agents are the rotaviruses, enterotoxigenic *Escherichia coli*, enteropathogenic *E. coli*, *Salmonella*, *Campylobacter jejuni*, *Vibrio cholerae*, *Shigella*, and *Cryptosporidium*.

Of these, the two most likely to cause fatal dehydration are rotavirus in children younger than 1 year of age and enterotoxigenic *E. coli* in children younger than 3 years. However, as far as the physician is concerned, it matters little what the causative agent is because few will respond to specific chemotherapy, and the treatment is the same for all.

Clinical Features

The attacks, of which there may be several each year, start acutely with watery diarrhea, the young child passing 3 to 20 greenish, liquid stools daily. This may be accompanied by low fever, vomiting, and colic. The diarrhea usually lasts about a week before clearing spontaneously. In the hot climates of the tropics, however, severe dehydration may alter a troublesome diarrhea into a fatal attack within 2 or 3 days.

Treatment

The key to management is the prevention of dehydration. As soon as the child begins to have diarrhea, mothers should administer appropriate oral solutions. A cupful of such a solution is given by bottle, cup, or spoon for every diarrheal stool. The child is also encouraged to drink water or fruit juice, and it is essential that breast feeding should be maintained irrespective of the severity of the diarrhea. A suitable fluid for oral and nasogastric use is a low-osmolality glucose-salt solution that contains in 1 liter of water: sodium chloride (table salt) 2.6 gm, sodium citrate (baking soda) 2.9 gm, potassium chloride 1.5 gm, and glucose (dextrose) 13.5 gm.

Water prepared after boiling rice with the addition of electrolytes is also effective, not only in restoring hydration but also in controlling diarrhea. Rice protein contains important amino acids, and the slow intraluminal digestion of rice starch allows for a slow liberation of glucose without producing an osmolar load. Severe dehydration demands, whenever possible, immediate referral to a medical unit for intravenous treatment.

Diarrhea rarely occurs in isolation in children in the tropics. Usually, it is a part of a complex pediatric picture that may also include malnutrition, multiparasitism, and malaria. WHO is promoting a comprehensive approach to the management of the sick child through an Integrated Management of Childhood Illnesses (IMCI) program. Specific guidelines for diagnosis, treatment, and prevention can be found on the WHO website noted in this book's references.

Pig Bel

Pig bel, or *Enteritis necroticans*, is a severe, often-fatal, gangrenous enteritis caused by the toxin of *Clostridium perfringens*, which is an organism commonly present in the intestine of pigs and also widely distributed in the soil. It may also be found in the intestine of healthy people, but the exotoxin is normally rapidly destroyed by pancreatic trypsin.

Pig bel was first described in Papua New Guinea, affecting children 1 to 7 days after a feast in which large quantities of pig meat and sweet potatoes were eaten. The affected children presented with severe abdominal pain and distension, vomiting, and sometimes bloody stools. Treatment of severely afflicted children was based on intestinal decompression, IV fluids, and chloramphenicol, but surgery involving resection of gangrenous bowel was often required.

The mortality rate ranged from 15% to 40%, and at autopsy, the stomach and small bowel are grossly dilated, the walls appearing ischemic and gangrenous. There may be widespread necrosis of the gut mucosa, and gram-positive bacilli are seen in the mucosa and submucosa. In addition to the large intake of organisms during the feast, previous malnutrition and the trypsin inhibitor present in the sweet potatoes may also be potentiating factors. This condition has now also been reported from Indonesia, Malaysia, Thailand, and Uganda. A satisfactory vaccine is now available.

Traveler's Diarrhea

Half of the tens of millions of North American and European tourists to the tropics each year suffer short attacks of diarrhea during their travels. The most notorious organisms involved are the Norwalk-like viruses and the enterotoxigenic *Escherichia coli* (ETEC), which resembles *Vibrio cholerae* in causing an adenylcyclase-induced enteropathy. Other pathogens reported as causing this condition include *Campylobacter jejuni*, multiple *Salmonella* serotypes, *Vibrio parahaemolyticus*, non-01 *Vibrio cholerae*, *Aeromonas hydrophila*, and *Plesiomonas shigellosis*.

Commonly on about the fourth day of the visit, there is a sudden onset of abdominal colic, followed by watery diarrhea with the passing of 3 to 8 liquid stools daily. The attacks usually last 1 to 3 days before resolving spontaneously, but may be sufficiently severe to temporarily confine the sufferer to bed, seriously restricting scheduled activities. In the great majority of these attacks, the only treatment required is a day in bed, fasting from all food, and taking plenty of fluids. Loperamide or bismuth subsalicylate may be helpful, but severe attacks may call for cotrimoxazole, doxycycline, ciprofloxin, or as resistance inevitably develops, one of the newer generation of antimicrobials.

Giardiasis

Giardia lambia, an enteric protozoan first described in frigid Russia, also causes human disease in warm and temperate climates. It is an extremely common infection, especially in children, in many parts of the tropics. Travelers may become infected and appear to develop more significant abdominal bloating, flatulence, and diarrhea. The incubation period is longer than with other forms of traveler's diarrhea, but the attacks are more persistent so that patients often present after their return home complaining of loss of weight and flatulence. Backpack travelers are particularly prone to infection. The pathogenesis of the diarrhea is not fully understood, but there may be malabsorptive features. The diagnosis is confirmed by finding cysts or trophozoites in the stools, or occasionally, in duodenal aspirates. Both forms of the protozoan have very distinctive appearances (cf., Figure 12). Treatment with metronidazole, albendazole, quinacrine hydrochloride (mepacrine), tinidazole, paromomycin—and, especially in children, nitazoxanide—is usually successful.

Tropical Enteropathy

This rather misleading term refers to a nonpathological state common throughout the tropics in which the structure and function of the small intestinal mucosa differs from that in temperate regions. When examined under the dissecting microscope, jejunal biopsies show leaves, ridges, or even convolutions, while histological sections display variations in villous architecture with prominent plasma cell infiltration. D-xylose absorption is also subnormal compared with Western standards. This is a physiological adaptation to a more luxuriant intestinal bacterial flora.

Tropical Sprue

In 1818, a young medical officer, George Ballingal, Surgeon to Her Majesty's 33rd Regiment of Foot in Bengal, described two contrasting forms of dysentery. The first was an acute disease in which the pathological changes were confined to the colon and that tended to affect soldiers soon after their arrival in India. The other type was a chronic condition known as the "hepatic flux," which affected men after they had been resident some time in India. It was characterized by urgent diarrhea with the passage of white frothy stools, multiple abdominal symptoms, and eventual debility and emaciation. The condition was well known to soldiers as the "white flux," and they were acquainted with its tedious and intractable nature. Martin (1856) recorded that patients with this condition, when evacuated home to Britain, suffered from anemia in its most aggravated form.

Tropical sprue has been defined as intestinal malabsorption occurring in the tropics for which no other cause can be found. Such a definition may well refer to a number of conditions, but the following account is of one very characteristic clinicopathological syndrome endemic in southeast Asia, India, and the Caribbean, but has also been recorded from southern Africa.

Pathology

During the first few weeks of the illness, the small intestinal mucosa may appear normal, or there may be increased cellular infiltration of the lamina propria with plasma cells and lymphocytes. Subsequently, the jejunal mucosa has either grossly swollen leaves, or more commonly, convolutions; microscopy reveals partial villous atrophy. There is intestinal malabsorption of fat, D-xylose, vitamin B12, and dietary folate, producing a progressive deficiency of folate and vitamin B12. After 4 to 5 months, a megaloblastic anemia due to folate deficiency develops; and after 3 to 5 years, a similar anemia due to vitamin B12 deficiency is seen. In patients previously deficient in these vitamins, the progress of both intestinal and hematological abnormalities is greatly accelerated.

Clinical Features

The onset may be with a sudden watery diarrhea, abdominal colic, and vomiting suggestive of an acute infection. The diarrhea will slowly change to that commonly seen in intestinal malabsorption.

In some patients, the onset is more gradual, and diarrhea may be mild or even nonexistent. Typically, the diarrhea is nocturnal or confined to the morning; defecation is urgent and usually preceded by colic and followed by relief. The stools are pale in color, of the consistency of porridge, with an extremely offensive odor. In other patients, the main complaint is of an intolerable loss of energy so that every effort becomes a burden. The appetite is deranged with patients either loathing the thought of food, or alternatively, feeling hungry but unable to take more than one or two mouthfuls. Weight is lost at a rate of about 15 pounds per month.

After 6 weeks, aphthous ulcers may appear on the oral mucosa followed later by a painful glossitis, stomatitis, and sometimes dysphagia. After 4 to 5 months, a varying degree of anemia can be found. By this time, patients may be severely ill with frequent vomiting, anorexia, and extreme fatigue and weakness. They lie curled up in bed, resisting any questioning in a manner similar to that seen in Addison's disease; this resemblance may be heightened by the presence of skin and oral pigmentation.

In yet other patients, it seems that the pathological process may remain subclinical for many years until they present with severe megaloblastic anemia mainly due to vitamin B12 deficiency. If treated with folic acid at this stage, they may develop subacute combined degeneration of the spinal cord. Fortunately, most are misdiagnosed as suffering from pernicious anemia and mistakenly receive appropriate therapy.

Diagnosis

A definitive diagnosis of tropical sprue can be made only by the demonstration of characteristic intestinal and hematological derangements related to a period of likely "infection." There must be malabsorption of fat, D-xylose, and vitamin B12 administered with intrinsic factor. A barium meal is required to exclude any anatomical defect; no abnormality will be seen in the first few months, but later, there is often dilatation of the jejunum with thickening of the transverse mucosal folds. Jejunal biopsies may be normal during the first few weeks, but by 3 months, there are usually convolutions with partial villous atrophy.

Serum folate is reduced from the start, and hypersegmentation of neutrophils occurs early. By 3 months, the bone marrow will show some megaloblastic change, and the red cell folate level will be reduced. After 4 to 5 months, a frank megaloblastic anemia due to folate deficiency develops. The serum vitamin B12 will be in the range of 90 to 200 ng per ml; after 3 to 4 years, the serum vitamin B12 is in the range seen in pernicious anemia. These temporal relationships will be greatly accelerated in the presence of previous folate deficiency. Thus patients developing sprue in late pregnancy or the puerperium develop severe intestinal change and severe anemia within 2 to 3 weeks. Associated iron deficiency is common in female patients, but vitamin D deficiency appears to be very uncommon. It is interesting that children, who rarely develop severe folate deficiency, also rarely develop sprue.

Treatment

Patients with sprue of less than 1 year's duration show a dramatic response to treatment with folic acid. The diarrhea ceases, the appetite becomes ravenous, the mouth heals; in the absence of iron deficiency, there is a full hematological response and a steady gain of weight. Following an initial increase in steatorrhea, probably due to the increased appetite, intestinal absorption of fat and D-xylose improve, and the jejunal mucosa also shows rapid healing. However, intestinal malabsorption of vitamin B12 may persist, the jejunal mucosa does not return to normal, and relapse is common. To obtain a complete cure, patients should be given 3 consecutive 5-day courses of oral broad-spectrum antibiotics; tetracycline and chloramphenicol are commonly used. Patients with chronic sprue also require vitamin B12.

The pathogenesis of tropical sprue remains unclear. For more than 100 years, authorities have debated whether it is an infectious or a deficiency disease; some of the following facts may be relevant. In many patients, the onset is associated with an acute infection, and the disease may be cured by treatment with oral broad-spectrum antibacterial drugs. Conditions that interfere with the normal jejunal flora and encourage coliform growth have been linked with outbreaks of sprue, and bacteriological studies have demonstrated chronic colonization of the jejunum with certain pathogenic coliforms. Sprue is not, however, a type of blind loop syndrome, because although vitamin B12 malabsorption may be rapidly corrected by antibiotics, this vitamin reaches the ileum normally as a complex with intrinsic factor. It is obvious, however, that there is a very close relationship between the folate and/ or vitamin B12 state of patients and the intestinal lesion in sprue. It is also clear that sprue may become epidemic in troops on a folate-deficient diet. Perhaps both infection and deficiency are involved in the etiology of this strange condition.

Miscellaneous Malabsorptive Syndromes

Tropical sprue is by no means the only form of intestinal malabsorption seen in the tropics. The first symptoms of adult celiac disease may occur during a sojourn in the tropics, and tuberculous enteritis in the indigenous population may very closely resemble sprue. Early *Strongyloides stercoralis* infection may also present as an acute malabsorption syndrome, and disseminated strongyloidiasis can cause a severe, protein-losing enteropathy with malabsorption. A rather similar condition is caused by *Capillaria philippinensis*. Alpha chain disease, rare in most parts of the world, is fairly frequent in the eastern Mediterranean and the Arabian peninsula. It is a severe enteropathy associated with finger clubbing and characterized by a heavy infiltration of the intestinal mucosa with plasma cells producing only heavy chain IgA. Diagnosis is important because it responds to long-term treatment with tetracycline, with or without cytotoxic drugs.

Finally, intestinal malabsorption due to chronic pancreatitis is common in parts of Africa, Indonesia, and southern India. Attacks of abdominal pain may start at ages 6 to 10 years; and by early adult life, diarrhea, steatorrhea, weight loss, and diabetes develops. Plain x-ray of the abdomen reveals pancreatic calcification.

Viral Infections of the Tropics

Several viral infections are important causes of severe disease in the tropics. Some of these viruses, such as those causing yellow fever, dengue, and Japanese B encephalitis, are now largely confined to the tropics. Others, such as the viruses of measles, hepatitis B, and the retroviruses, although occurring worldwide, pose special problems in the tropics.

The Arboviruses

Arthropod-borne, or arboviruses, are important causes of short-term fevers, encephalitis, hepatitis, and hemorrhagic fevers. Most are maintained in nature as animal infections, and all are transmitted by blood-sucking insects: mainly, mosquitoes or ticks. The viruses multiply in the insects and can be transmitted only following a period of "extrinsic incubation," usually lasting about 10 days. As transovarial viral infection is common in these insects, they also function as important reservoir hosts.

Most of the vertebrate hosts for arboviruses are animals to which the organisms have become well adapted. Apart from viremia, they rarely show evidence of disease. Man is an irregular host, and although the majority of human infections are subclinical or of a relatively mild nature, others result in severe and even fatal disease. The arboviruses have been classified into a number of groups on the basis of the inhibition agglutination test of Casals.

Yellow Fever

Carlos J. Finlay, a Cuban physician, suggested in 1881 that yellow fever was carried by the mosquito *Stegomia fasciata (Aedes aegypti)*. The

United States, forced by epidemics of yellow fever that annually threatened the Mississippi valley and delayed the construction of the Panama
Canal, appointed an Army Investigative Board in 1900 consisting of
Drs. Reed, Carrol, Agramonte, and Lazear, now famous names in the
history of tropical medicine. By 1903, the Board had demonstrated that
infection was indeed caused by a submicroscopic agent transmitted by
Aedes aegypti.

The importance of this finding was confirmed when control of the
mosquito resulted in a dramatic cessation of yellow fever. During the
course of this investigation, Carrol and Lazear had allowed themselves
to be bitten by mosquitoes, which had previously fed on patients with
yellow fever. Both men contracted the disease, and Lazear died. Misfor-
tune did not end there because their studies were mercilessly—and
inaccurately—attacked, and Reed, like Chagas, suffered an early death.
"Yellow Jack" continues to take a heavy toll of lives among the rural
inhabitants of the Guinea savanna lands of West Africa, where it
remains endemic and epidemic. Table 6 shows some tropical arboviruses causing significant human disease.

Pathology

The yellow fever virus is a spherical Group B arbovirus transmitted to
man by *Aedes* and *Haemogogus* mosquitoes after an extrinsic period
of 9 to 12 days. This development phase requires an environmental
temperature exceeding 70°F. In man, the viremia is brought to an
abrupt end after 4 days with the appearance of antibodies.

The main target of infection is the liver, which is affected by midzonal necrosis of hepatocytes Acidophilic round masses of hyaline material, known as "Councilman bodies," form in affected cells.
Intranuclear inclusions—Torres bodies—are also histologic findings.
Fatty change occurs, but there is little or no inflammatory cell reaction,
and the hepatic reticulum framework is preserved. Following recovery,
liver structure rapidly returns to normal.

Clinical Features

The severity of an attack of yellow fever varies greatly. In the more
severely affected patients, after an incubation period of 3 to 6 days,

Table 6. Some tropical arboviruses causing significant human disease

Group Virus	Disease	Distribution
A		
Chikungunya	Dengue-like	East Africa, India
O'nyong nyong	Dengue-like	East Africa
Igbo-Ora	Dengue-like	West Africa
Venezuelan equine	Encephalitis	South America, Central America
Ross River	Epidemic polyarthritis	Australia, South Pacific
B		
West Nile	Dengue-like, encephalitis	Africa, southeast Asia, North America
Wesselbron	Dengue-like	Africa, Thailand
Dengue	Dengue	Most of tropics
Yellow fever	Hepatitis, hemorrhagic fever	Africa, North America, Central America
Kyasanur Forest	Hemorrhagic fever	Southern India
Japanese B	Encephalitis	South Asia, Indonesia, Philippines
Murray Valley	Encephalitis	New Guinea, Australia
Ungrouped		
Rift Valley fever	Hemorrhagic fever	Africa
Sandfly fever	Dengue-like	Mediterranean, Middle East

there is a sudden onset of fever, chills, severe headache, muscular pains, epigastric pain, and often vomiting. The face is flushed, conjunctivae injected, tongue coated, and the breath foul. The pulse rate is at first rapid and then falls away, so that there is a relative bradycardia (Faget's sign). After 3 or 4 days, there may be some remission lasting a few hours to a day, but then the patient can deteriorate rapidly.

Jaundice, which may have been mild, now intensifies, and congestion gives place to bleeding with purpura, swollen gums, epistaxis, hematemesis, and melena. There is increasing prostration with hypotension, oliguria, or anuria; the urine being thick, cloudy, laden with bile, and, on heating, forming an almost-solid mass. The serum bilirubin and transaminases are high, but the alkaline phosphatase remains normal. There may be hypoglycemia, acidosis, and a rapidly

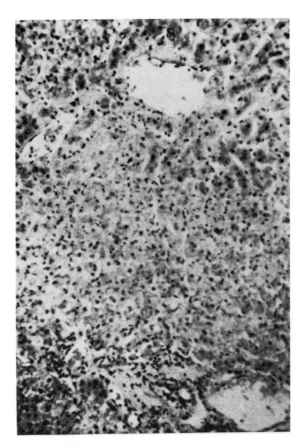

FIGURE 22: Postmortem liver from an African man
demonstrating marked midzonal necrosis of yellow fever.

rising blood urea. Patients usually remain conscious and rational, but
there may be periods of mental confusion and delirium. Death is usually preceded by stupor and coma. The fatality rate in the severe form
of yellow fever is about 50%, but if the patient survives until the tenth
day, full recovery can be expected.

In single, and especially in mild, infections, a clinical diagnosis may
not be possible, and yellow fever is usually considered only when an
outbreak of hepatitis is associated with a sudden, dramatic mortality.
Laboratory confirmation is based on virus isolation, demonstration of
specific IgM antibodies to yellow fever virus by capture enzyme linked

immunosorbent assay, and gene amplification. There is no specific chemotherapy available, and treatment can be only supportive. Intensive
care units and skills may substantially reduce the mortality rate, but
such facilities are seldom available in endemic areas. There has been
an effort, therefore, to establish mobile units equipped with diagnostic
and advanced treatment facilities.

Epidemiology

A primary cycle of yellow fever infection is present in tropical rain
forests where transmission occurs between canopy monkeys and mosquitoes, but human yellow fever is seldom seen there. Recent African
epidemics have all occurred in the Guinea-savannah area, at the edges
of the so-called "emergence zones," where nonimmunes are first
exposed. Here, following rains in the gallery forest, a high density of
infected, tree hole–breeding mosquitoes feed on a nonimmune population. Monkeys play a part in this setting; various species raid agricultural adjoining land and help to transmit sylvatic yellow fever.

In Central America and South America, a similar cycle exists, involving howler monkeys and *Haemogogus* mosquitoes, but human infection
is limited to sporadic cases of yellow fever among men working or
traveling in the forest.

In urban yellow fever, humans are the hosts responsible for circulation of virus together with the domestic vector *Aedes aegypti*. Uncontrolled urbanization and the presence of abundant *Aedes aegypti* vectors
constitute a dangerous situation. Epidemics of urban yellow fever result
from the introduction of virus, usually by humans traveling from
endemic rural areas. The fatality rate is high. Recent epidemics have
occurred in various west African countries. Urban yellow fever has been
controlled in Central and South America, but the danger of reintroduc-
tion still exists, especially in cities near jungle areas.

Vaccination is the best way of controlling yellow fever. A thermosta-
ble 17D vaccine is now available, which protects for 10 years. Mass
vaccination campaigns have been undertaken, and in some countries,
yellow fever vaccine has been incorporated in the Expanded Programme of Immunization (EPI) together with measles vaccine. Yellow
fever vaccine should not be given to infants younger than 1 year of age

nor to pregnant women. Severe neurotropic and hepatotoxic reactions, although rare, are reported.

Dengue Fever

The dengue fever virus is a very small togovirus containing a single strand of RNA enclosed in a tight envelope. Four strains are recognized. The virus can be cultured only with difficulty; mosquito cell monolayers are used for this purpose, and the strains are identified by serological reactions. There is no known natural animal reservoir of infection, and the virus is conveyed from man to man by *Aedes* mosquitoes.

Clinical Features

The incubation period is 4 to 6 days, during which the virus multiplies in lymph nodes. This is followed by a viremia lasting 2 to 4 days, clearing with the appearance of IgM and later IgG antibodies. In the "typical case," the onset is sudden with chills, fever, severe frontal and retro-orbital headache, and myalgic pains ("breakbone fever"). Other symptoms may include abdominal pain and vomiting, and cough is particularly common in children. The face is flushed, the eyes congested, and there may be lymph node and liver enlargement. The fever lasts about 1 week, but is interrupted on the third or fourth day when the temperature falls to normal for 24 hours, the so-called "saddle back fever." The pulse rate tends to be disproportionately slow, especially during the second phase, when a maculopapular rash may develop. The diagnosis is made on epidemiological and clinical grounds: by isolation of the virus, serological tests, and detection of dengue virus antigen and dengue virus RNA. Treatment can be only supportive.

Epidemiology

Dengue is endemic in southeast Asia, where most of the indigenous population are infected in childhood, when the disease is mild or subclinical. The chief vector is *Aedes aegypti*, a peridomestic mosquito, but *Aedes albopictus* is an important vector in rural areas. Dengue is now known to be endemic in many parts of Africa and recurrent epidemics occur in the Caribbean, Central America, and South America.

Hemorrhagic Fevers

The term "hemorrhagic fever" is given to a clinicopathological syndrome, which can be caused by certain arboviruses, as well as by other zoonotic viruses that are not transmitted by arthropods. It seems likely that the pathological features arise from a violent immunological reaction to the virus with release of chemical mediators, causing widespread capillary damage and increased capillary permeability. Loss of plasma fluid into the tissues results in hypovolemia. At the same time, a consumptive coagulopathy with thrombocytopenia develops. In addition, many—if not all these infections—are associated with a form of hepatitis characterized by focal eosinophilic necrosis of hepatocytes, little or no inflammatory reaction, and reduced synthesis of various coagulation factors. Another common feature is the frequency of nosocomial and laboratory infections, which tend to be severe.

Dengue Hemorrhagic Fever (DHF)

This dangerous illness may occur when an individual possessing antibodies from a previous dengue infection is reinfected with a different strain of dengue virus. The immunologic response, instead of being with IgM, is an anamnestic reaction with IgG antibodies persisting from the initial infection. These antibodies combine with the new strain to form immune complexes that, attaching to macrophages and monocytes, further facilitate entry of the virus into these cells. Massive viral replication then occurs, and these heavily infected cells become the targets for an immune elimination response, resulting in the release of chemical mediators of capillary damage, with a massive increase in vascular permeability. This form of dengue is seen predominantly in children and occasionally in infants 3 to 6 months old in whom dengue antibodies received from the mother have persisted. Infections in adults also occur.

Clinical Features

During the first 3 to 4 days, the illness is indistinguishable from uncomplicated dengue of the mild type, but then the child becomes seriously ill: light-headed, restless, irritable, sweating, and increasingly prostrated.

The four grades of DHF are as follows:

Grade 1: Platelets <100,000 + positive tourniquet test
Grade 2: Platelets <100,000 + spontaneous bleeding
Grade 3: Platelets <100,000 + shock, BP <200 mm Hg
Grade 4: Platelets <100,000 + unrecordable pulse and BP

The diagnosis is usually clear from the clinical manifestations. Treatment is directed against the shock and hemorrhage rather than against the infection. The hemocrit is often raised due to hemoconcentration, and there may be a false, and confusing, leukocytosis. Serological testing will reveal high titers of IgG. Bleeding is treated by infusion of platelet-rich fresh blood, and shock is treated by restoring the plasma volume with crystalloids or colloids. Oxygen is also indicated. However, special care must be taken during the early recovery phase not to overload the circulation, or the patient will develop acute pulmonary edema.

Epidemiology

Hemorrhagic dengue was first described from the Philippines in 1953, and during the 1960s, large outbreaks occurred in the cities of southeast Asia with thousands of deaths. Later, a large outbreak occurred in Cuba, when an epidemic of dengue 1 was followed 4 years later by an epidemic of dengue 2, affecting people of all ages.

Other tropical arboviruses causing hemorrhagic fever include the Crimean-Congo and the Kyasanur Forest, viruses both of which are transmitted from wild animals to man by ticks. Rift Valley fever virus is also an arbovirus, transmitted by culicine mosquitoes. This last infection was thought to be carried in camels from Sudan into Egypt, where, in 1977 and 1978, it caused large epidemics of a severe hemorrhagic fever. The main manifestations were hepatitis, encephalitis, and retinal vasculitis. Sheep, goats, and cattle were first affected, and transmission was by *Culex pipiens*. Humans were infected while handling infected meat. Recent epidemics have occurred in the southwest region of Saudi Arabia and Yemen.

Several other viruses, all of which primarily infect rodents, may cause human hemorrhagic fever. They are not arboviruses because they are not transmitted by insects. Table 7 shows epidemiology of some hemorrhagic fevers.

Lassa Fever

This virus, like those causing hemorrhagic fever in South America, is an arenovirus related to the etiologic agent of lymphocytic choriomeningitis. It grows well on Vero cell cultures. Under the electron microscope, it appears as a spherical particle containing "sandy granules." The usual mode of infection is by ingesting food contaminated with infected rat urine or saliva.

Clinical Features

The incubation period is usually 7 to 10 days, but unlike other hemorrhagic fevers, the onset is insidious with gradually rising fever, chills, malaise, anorexia, headache, and generalized aching. A characteristic feature toward the end of the first week is a sore throat with the appearance of white patches on the soft palate, tonsillar pillars, or pharyngeal mucosa, and these may be followed by enlargement of cervical lymph nodes and swelling of the face and neck.

As with other hemorrhagic fevers, the more dangerous period is during the second week, when increasing prostration can progress to

Table 7. Epidemiology of some hemorrhagic fevers

Virus	Distribution	Animal reservoir
Lassa fever virus	West Africa	*Mastomys natalensis*
Junin virus	Argentina	Field mice
Machupo virus	Bolivia	Mice
Hantan virus	Southeast Asia, Korea	Field mice, domestic rats
Ebola virus and Marburg virus	Congo, Sudan, Uganda, Angola	Not known

peripheral circulatory and renal failure, the most common causes of death. Pulmonary manifestations may simulate pneumonia. Hemorrhage is usually mild, limited to epistaxis, purpura, hemoptysis, or bleeding from needle puncture sites. The white cell count and the erythrocyte sedimentation rate (ESR) vary widely and are not helpful. The serum transaminases are always raised, and a value <3 times normal suggests a severe attack. Infection in pregnancy often leads to abortion, stillbirth, or death of the child immediately after birth. Infection in infancy may be manifest as a "swollen baby syndrome," with widespread edema, abdominal distension, and bleeding. Deafness is a late complication in 30% of patients.

A clinical diagnosis during the first week may be difficult; and in West Africa, where fever, sore throat, and pneumonia are common, the diagnosis is usually first suspected in patients with a fever for 7 consecutive days that does not respond to chloroquine or antibiotics. The virus may be demonstrated in the blood during the first few days, and by IgM antibodies from the fifth day. Antigen detection ELISA has proved very useful with positive samples obtained within 48 hours of admission.

The earlier mode of therapy with convalescent serum has now been superceded by treatment with ribavirin, which if given during the first week, reduces the mortality in severe cases from 55% to 5%.

Epidemiology

In spite of the nosocomial incidents that first drew attention to this disease, person-to-person infection is rare. Intensive care facilities may be required for severely ill patients, and treatment should not be compromised for fear of infection. In West Africa, where only serologically positive staff were used, whenever possible, to care for these patients, rudimentary isolation techniques were found sufficient to prevent spread of infection in hospital. Following a needle-stick accident, ribavirin taken for 10 days has proved an excellent prophylactic.

Lassa fever is now known to be common in several parts of rural or semi-rural west Africa. The virus is shed in the urine and saliva of small semi-domestic rats that abound in mud and thatch houses, and the source of most human infections is thought to be contaminated, stored grain. In these circumstances, the great majority of infections remain subclinical, and as many as 6% of the population of endemic areas acquire antibodies to the virus each year. Clinical disease is sporadic, and person-to-person infection is uncommon. Rats of the genus *Mastomys* are the natural hosts of Lassa virus; they are chronically infected and sustain long-term viremia.

Argentine Hemorrhagic Fever

This infection is due to the Junin virus, closely resembling Lassa fever. The infection is found primarily in field mice, which excrete the virus in urine. Human infections are mainly in maize harvesters, who are presumed to have inhaled the virus from dried excretions.

Hantan Virus

The Hantan group of viruses first came to worldwide attention when large numbers of United Nations troops in Korea developed a hemorrhagic fever complicated by severe renal involvement. This infection is now being recognized throughout southeast Asia and in the southwestern parts of the United States. The epidemiology appears to be similar to that of Argentine hemorrhagic fever, with natural infection occurring both in field mice and domestic rats.

Ebola and Marburg Virus Diseases

Two further bizarre-shaped, long filamentous viruses (filoviruses) cause hemorrhagic fever in Africa: the Ebola and Marburg viruses. The former gave rise to two large epidemics of severe hemorrhagic fever in southern Sudan and neighboring Congo, respectively, and recently in Uganda. Marburg caused a major outbreak in 2005 in Uganda and Angola. The epidemiology of these two virus infections remains obscure, but the devastating Congo epidemic was largely spread through the use of unsterilized needles and syringes.

The incubation period for Ebola virus is about 10 days. The onset is abrupt and nonspecific with fever, myalgia, severe headache, and extreme malaise. The appearance of a severe sore throat, chest and abdominal pain, vomiting, and a history of exposure should help to differentiate from other common fevers, such as malaria, typhoid, and so on. A papular rash on the trunk and back may occur, while the presence of vomiting and onset of mucosal bleeding are bad prognostic signs. Bleeding occurs the fifth day of illness with hematemesis, melena, epistaxis, and hemorrhage from the vagina. Infection in pregnancy is often fatal to both mother and fetus. There is a profound lymphopenia and elevation of liver enzymes. Treatment is symptomatic. Two new experimental vaccines for Marburg and Ebola have shown promising results in monkey trials.

Crimean-Congo Hemorrhagic Fever (CCHF)

This disease was first described in persons bitten by ticks while harvesting crops in the Crimean peninsula. The incubation period is short, only 1 to 3 days. Symptoms include fever, rigors, severe headache, myalgia, vomiting, and diarrhea. A petechial rash followed by the appearance of large bruises and ecchymoses occur in the first week of the illness. Bleeding from various orifices is common. Virus isolation and seroconversion confirm the diagnosis. Treatment is supportive.

Japanese B Encephalitis

This is one of the most important viral infections of rural Asia, where several strains of this avian virus are transmitted to man by culicine mosquitoes, with pigs often acting as amplifying hosts. Like dengue, the virus is a Group B arbovirus that first multiplies in lymph nodes before emerging as a viremia. Unfortunately, it can also enter the central nervous system (CNS), causing a meningoencephalitis marked by congestion, edema, focal hemorrhages, neuron degeneration, and demyelination. These changes are most severe in the thalamic region.

Clinical Features

The onset is with fever, soon followed by signs of encephalitis. Patients become either drowsy or irritable with severe headache and insomnia at night. This is often followed by a flattening of the affect, the face becoming mask-like, and the speech thick and slurred. There may be some neck stiffness, pupillary abnormality, nystagmus, ocular palsy, and tremor of the tongue and hands. Variable paresis may develop. Finally, the patient lapses into a stupor, and ultimately, into a coma with decerebrate rigidity. The mortality rate varies from 20% to 65%, but the outcome is difficult to assess, and even patients in deep coma can recover. If the patient survives, there is usually complete amnesia concerning the illness, but convalescence is very slow, and residual neurological and psychiatric defects are not uncommon.

The diagnosis is usually made on clinical and epidemiological grounds. Cerebral malaria and other forms of meningitis must be excluded. While the cerebrospinal fluid is clear, it usually is under increased pressure, and the white blood cell (WBC) ranges from 20 to 100 per mm^3. The virus may be isolated from the cerebrospinal fluid (CSF) or from the brain after death. The diagnosis is usually confirmed by isolation of virus, a rise in specific antibodies between acute and convalescent sera, and detection of virus antigen or RNA. IgM antibodies appear in the serum and CSF early in the disease, and can be detected by ELISA or rapid diagnostic kits. Computerized tomography (CT) or magnetic resonance imaging (MRI) shows characteristic midbrain changes. Treatment can be only supportive; skillful nursing is particularly important, and respiratory assistance may be required. Hyperpyrexia is a particular problem.

Epidemiology

Birds, particularly herons, disseminate infection, but probably the main reservoir is mosquitoes. In regions where there is little change in climate throughout the year, infection remains endemic and sporadic, but in other areas, annual epidemics occur at the period of greatest mosquito activity. The vectors include several species of culicine mosquitoes; the most notorious is *Culex tritaeniorrhyncus*, which is a mosquito that breeds in rice fields. Pigs are readily infected, maintain a chronic viremia, and are important amplifying hosts. Control measures include the use of residual insecticides in houses and outhouses, as well as the vaccination of pigs and their segregation from human habitations. Two vaccines for human use are available: a Chinese, live-attenuated vaccine and a formalin-inactivated vaccine.

Viral Hepatitis in the Tropics

Viral hepatitis with jaundice in the tropics may be caused by yellow fever virus, Rift Valley fever virus, cytomegalovirus, and the Epstein-Barr virus (EBV), but the term "viral hepatitis" usually refers to infections with hepatitis A virus (HAV), hepatitis B virus (HBV), hepatitis C virus (HCV), the delta virus (HDV) and the hepatitis E virus (HEV). HAV, an enterovirus, is of little importance to the indigenous population of the tropics. Infection in childhood is almost universal, mainly subclinical, and is followed by lasting immunity. However, visitors from other regions, where improvement in sanitation has greatly reduced infections in youth, are liable to overt acute hepatitis. Hepatitis is the most common medical reason for evacuation of Peace Corps workers from the tropics and is almost universal in Western missionaries; for example, after a decade living with indigenous populations, almost 100% of missionaries studied had HAV antibodies. Temporary protection may be given to travelers to endemic areas by intramuscular (IM) inoculation with pooled immunoglobulin or by use of an inactivated viral vaccine. Long-lasting protection can now be realized by administration of two injections, six months apart, of the inactivated viral vaccine.

HBV, HCV, and HDV infections are, in contrast, causes of severe disease. HBV and HCV often results in chronic active hepatitis and can cause primary hepatoma. Early therapy with interferon and ribavarin can prevent this fatal development. Both HDV and HEV have been associated with epidemics in the tropics and lead to significant mortality.

Hepatitis B Virus

HBV infection in the tropics is almost as universal as HAV and also occurs at an early age, either at birth or in early childhood. At this age, the immune response of the body is immature, the virus is not eliminated, and 90% of these infants or young children become chronic carriers. By early adult life, this carrier state is cleared in all but 5% to 20%, but persistent carriers can develop chronic hepatitis and primary carcinoma of the liver. It has been estimated that a total of two billion people worldwide have been infected with the hepatitis B virus, with more than 350 million suffering from chronic liver infections. Hepatitis B is endemic in China and other parts of Asia. In southeast Asia, many of these carriers have been infected in the perinatal period, most acquiring their disease from HBe Ag–positive mothers. In Africa, on the other hand, most infections occur at the preschool age and are acquired from other children by close contact. Early childhood infection is usually marked by a high titer of HBs Ag and HBe Ag, so that these children are highly infective.

Clinical Features

Hepatitis in adult carriers may be either of the chronic persistent or the chronic active varieties. The former is usually not associated with significant symptoms, but if these individuals are HBe Ag–positive, they may still progress to cirrhosis. Chronic active hepatitis is a relapsing condition of varied severity, but throughout the tropics, it differs from the autoimmune form seen in Europe and the United States in that treatment with corticosteroids, although offering transient relief, tends to lead to early relapse and increased mortality. Progress to a coarse macro-lobular cirrhosis is common and accounts for the high prevalence of cirrhosis of the liver among African and southern Asia populations. After a time, the HBV genome may integrate with the host hepatocyte genome. The hepatocytes continue to secrete HBs Ag, but core markers are no longer produced, and HBe Ag is no longer detected in the serum. Clones of hepatocytes containing integrated HBV genome form the basis of malignant transformation, resulting in hepatocellular carcinoma.

These are large tumors consisting of bizarre columns of neoplastic cells, caricatures of normal liver cells, that are surrounded by blood spaces resembling liver sinusoids, with a special tendency to rupture. The condition runs a fulminating course, with the mean survival time of 11 weeks from the onset of symptoms and 6 weeks from diagnosis to death. The surgical resectability rate is less than 1%, and prolongation of survival can seldom be achieved by chemotherapy. Diagnosis is relatively simple, as these malignant cells secrete large amounts of alpha fetoprotein, and the serum level of this substance will exceed 800 mg per ml.

Chemotherapy is of little value, but we do have the means to prevent it. Although the virus cannot be grown, a very effective vaccine has been produced from the plasma of carriers by separating the outer envelope of the virus (HBs Ag), which is immunogenic but noninfectious, from the infectious inner core. Three doses of the vaccines are given IM 2 to 3 months apart with a booster dose after 1 year. The ideal is that all susceptible people living in regions of high endemicity should be vaccinated.

In southeast Asia, where infection is often perinatal, vaccination should commence at birth; in Africa, vaccination should commence at 3 months and be integrated with other prophylactic immunizations. Newborn children of HBe Ag–positive mothers should also be given hepatitis B immune globulin (HBIG) in a dose of 0.5 ml IM. Further prevention can be realized by screening all HBs Ag–positive adults for raised serum alpha fetoprotein concentrations; these titers rise up to 2 years before the first symptoms of hepatoma appear, and resection at that time is a comparatively simple affair. The main problems concerning mass vaccination arise from the cost and limited availability of the vaccines. However, new vaccines based on DNA-recombinant technology are now becoming available, and it is hoped that these will be less expensive and be produced in unlimited amounts.

Another closely related hepatavirus, HBV2, has been reported as causing a carrier state in west Africa. Infected individuals are HBs Ag–positive, but anti–HBc-negative. Following cessation of the carrier state, anti-HBs does not appear, and these individuals are not protected from infection with HBV1. It is not certain whether this virus is associated with hepatic disease, but it may account for many individuals who have both HBs Ag and anti-HBs in their serum.

Deltavirus

The deltavirus is a defective RNA organism that can replicate only when encapsulated with the surface envelope of HBV (HBs Ag).

Infection can be maintained in only those individuals whose liver cells produce HBs Ag. It is transmitted in a similar way to HBV, and coinfection can occur. The importance of this infection in the tropics stems from the enormous numbers of HBs Ag carriers. Superinfection with deltavirus may result in one of the following:

Cessation of the carrier state

A chronic, fulminant hepatitis

A chronic carrier state with persisting HBV and HDV, which is associated with a worse prognosis

This carrier state is suggested by the finding of both HBs Ag and a high titer of anti-HDV in the serum.

Retroviral Infections in the Tropics

Human Immune-Deficiency Virus Type I (HIV1)

During the last two decades of the twentieth century, Acquired Immune-Deficiency Syndrome (AIDS), utterly changed the nature of medicine in the tropics. From the brothels of southeast Asia, in the barrios of Latin America, along the highways and commerce lanes of Africa, and around the world, AIDS exploded. The AIDS epidemic spread with such fury that it became the leading cause of death in Africa, far exceeding malaria and tuberculosis combined.

By the end of the first decade of the twenty-first century, more than 33 million people worldwide had HIV/AIDS; two-thirds of that number were in sub-Saharan Africa, and another 20% were in Asia and the Pacific. Infection rates of 30% of the adult population have been reported in some African areas. Therapeutic advances in developed countries were too expensive for the paltry health budgets of most tropical nations. The cost of AIDS also overwhelmed traditional public health programs that might have been devoted to other preventable illnesses. Furthermore, AIDS influenced the clinical presentation and incidence of all other infections in the tropics.

The disease is transmitted by sexual contact; blood contamination; or during birth from infected mother to child. The ease of transmission is influenced by many factors, but the most important is the level of viremia. The HIV virus contains a unique reverse–transcriptase enzyme that allows the RNA virus to make a DNA copy and invade and replicate in human helper T-cell lymphocytes, leading to a collapse of the immune system.

Following infection with HIV, serum antibodies may be detected by ELISA after 4 to 7 weeks, but most patients do not serologically convert for 2 to 4 months. The virus contains core proteins and envelope glyco-proteins that can be separated by electrophoresis. When these are exposed to patient's sera on nitrocellulose strips, specific bands of a characteristic profile develop (Western blot). The main target cells are the CD4 (T4) helper lymphocytes. These cells play a key role in the immunological responses to infection. After a latent period, which may extend to years, a quantitative and qualitative defect in these cells develops although precisely how this is mediated is unclear. As a result, the individual suffers from an increased susceptibility to opportunistic, often latent, infections and to certain malignant tumors, possibly of viral origin. Other target cells include macrophages related to neuro-glial and other glial cells, the follicular dentritic cells of the germinal centers of lymph nodes, and possibly certain enterocytes.

Clinical Features

The clinical picture of HIV infection is extremely diverse. Some patients may remain asymptomatic, but infectious, for many years. HIV infection progresses to AIDS when patients' CD4 cells levels fall precip-itously, viremia rises, and opportunistic infections or specific tumors develop. Early in the course, most AIDS victims note loss of weight and energy.

Seroconversion may be accompanied by a glandular fever–like syn-drome with or without a transient encephalopathy or other neurologi-cal manifestations. This is then usually followed by a long latent period that may last several years. In African patients, the onset of AIDS tends to follow a characteristic pattern. including persistent nonbloody diar-rhea, generalized weakness, and constant or intermittent fever, often accompanied by a cough and a pruritic generalized rash. Common opportunistic infections include candidiasis that may affect the esopha-gus, causing dysphagia; herpes simplex, which may result in perianal ulceration; recurrent herpes zoster; cytomegalovirus, and JC virus reactivation. Diarrhea is often caused by *Entamoeba histolytica*, *Cryptosporidium*, or *Isospora belli* infection. Common complications in Africa are tuberculosis, cryptococcal infection, and Kaposi's sarcoma.

It is estimated that about one-half of the adult population in the age group most likely to be HIV1-infected also harbor *Mycobacterium tuberculosis* organisms that reactivate when cell-mediated immune defenses decline. It is, therefore, not surprising that so many African AIDS patients show evidence of active pulmonary tuberculosis (TB). The pathological lesions tend to resemble those of primary TB, being multibacillary with prominent necrosis, while granuolmata and lymphocytes are usually absent or sparse. Chest x-rays reveal enlarged hilar nodes, with or without pulmonary infiltration seen in the middle or lower zones, and sparing of the apices. Cavitation is rare. Infection tends to disseminate, and the tuberculin test is often negative.

Cryptococcal infection was by no means rare in Africa, but the increased prevalence of this fungal infection was one of the first indications of the prevalence of HIV1 in the Congo. In AIDS patients, the infection may remain relatively silent, but a common presentation of this complication is subacute meningoencephalitis. The diagnosis is best confirmed by the demonstration of spores in the CSF with Indian ink preparations.

Kaposi's sarcoma has long been endemic in central Africa, where it accounted for 9% of all malignant tumors. It was formerly seen in men older than age 40, presenting as purple, hyperpigmented nodules or plaques on the periphery of the limbs. Progress was slow, remission not uncommon, and lesions responded well to treatment with radiotherapy or cytotoxic drugs. In 1983, an atypical form of this condition began to be seen first in Zambia.

Younger adults presented with generalized symmetrical lymph node enlargement, and biopsies revealed the spindle-shaped cells with blood spaces characteristic of Kaposi's sarcoma. Other patients presented with raspberry-like tumors in the mouth. On endoscopy, they could be found in the esophagus, stomach, and rectum. Skin lesions often involved the trunk; if they affected the limbs, they tended to be associated with severe edema. Although there might be an initial response to radiation, these patients quickly relapsed and died within a few months.

It was soon recognized that this aggressive form of Kaposi's sarcoma in adults was a manifestation of AIDS. In Africa, 15% of AIDS victims have Kaposi's sarcoma; the incidence in the homosexual AIDS population in the United States is higher.

In a condition in which particular organs may be affected by several major pathogens, and in a region where medical facilities are limited, it is clearly difficult to be dogmatic about the prevalence of the various opportunistic complications. Severe amebiasis and disseminated *Strongyloides* infection are well documented. It does seem, however, that certain infections common in American and European AIDS are uncommon or rare in African patients. These include *Pneumocystis carinii*, *M. avium intracellulare*, and perhaps *Toxoplasma* infection. It is surprising that there appears to be no association between AIDS and severe *P. falciparum* malaria, except in pregnant women, nor has there been an increase in the incidence of the prevalent B cell tumor, Burkitt's lymphoma.

Diagnosis and Therapy

The clinical diagnosis of HIV1 infection is particularly difficult in African children. They present with fever, diarrhea, anemia, pneumonia, lymphadenopathy, dermatitis, thrush, and malnutrition, all common features in African pediatric practice. Diagnostic ELISA or Western Blot HIV kits are highly accurate and available.

Therapy is constantly evolving, and the various "cocktails" of viral inhibitors have now made a uniformly fatal disease a chronic infection. The major problem in most tropical countries is the cost of current drug regimens. Therapeutic regimens for AIDS using commercial pharmaceuticals cost more than $15,000 US per year, a sum that is impossible for a developing nation's health budget. Some poor nations, led by the example of Brazil, have successfully secured the right to supercede drug patent restrictions in order to manufacture low-priced drugs to save their people. With excellent medical care and modern multidrug "cocktails," HIV/AIDS has become a chronic illness in Western developed countries. The same cannot be said for the developing nations, especially in Africa. At present, there is no prophylactic nor therapeutic vaccine although animal research continues to offer promise.

Human Immune-Deficiency Virus Type 2 (HIV2)

Another retrovirus causing AIDS occurs in west Africa. This virus is more closely related to the simian T lymphotropic virus type III (STLV III) than to HIV1. It is transmitted in a similar manner. Cross-reactions occur with HIV1 in ELISA antihuman-immunoglobulin type assays, but not in competitive type assays. Commercial assay kits using HIV2 antigen are not readily available, but further confirmation is possible by Western blot. Another closely related retrovirus HTLV4 is also reported from this region.

Human T Lymphotropic Virus Type 1 (HTLV1)

This was the first human lymphotropic virus to be recognized and is endemic in the Japanese islands around Okinawa, among Japanese immigrants in Hawaii, in Papua New Guinea, in the Caribbean, and to a lesser extent in west Africa. It is not clear how infection is naturally transmitted, but mother to young child and conjugal infections do occur. The virus can also be transmitted in blood transfusions. The great majority of those infected remain free from overt disease, but a minority, after a period of often many years, will develop acute adult T-cell leukemia or a HTLV1-associated myelopathy (HAM).

Clinical Features

Theleukemia, in which malignant transformation of CD4 lymphocytes occurs, runs an aggressive course. The affected lymphocytes display a bizarre morphology, and hypercalcemia is a feature. Despite intensive chemotherapy, the survival time is less than 1 year.

The myelopathy consists of involvement of the pyramidal tracts by a lesion rather similar to that seen in multiple sclerosis. There is a slowly progressive spastic paraplegia. Sphincters are affected only late, and sensory disturbance is minimal. Lumbar puncture yields a clear fluid with a mild rise in protein, lymphocytes, and IgG immunoglobulin. The diagnosis is confirmed by the demonstration of specific antibodies in the serum and CSF by ELISA and Western blot. The response to treatment by corticosteroids is usually poor.

Intestinal Nematode Infections

Human intestinal infection with helminths is widespread in the tropics. According to a 2005 report by the World Health Organization (WHO), approximately one billion humans have ascariasis, and there are approximately 700 million cases of trichuriasis and hookworm infections worldwide. Most infections are light or moderate and do little to impair the health of the hosts, except in children, but heavy infection may result in clinical disease, and massive infections may be lethal. Convincing evidence now exists that geohelminths cause growth retardation and reduced learning ability in children.

Ascariasis

Ascaris lumbricoides is the roundworm most commonly found in man. Although most infections are asymptomatic, massive infection in children can cause intestinal obstruction, and invasion of the biliary and pancreatic ducts may lead to cholangitis, liver abscess, or pancreatitis.

The Parasite

The adult worms are white, creamy, or pink in color. They are the largest of the intestinal nematodes, the females measuring 20 to 35 cm and the males 15 to 30 cm in length. They live free in the small intestine where the female lays up to 200,000 eggs daily. These eggs have a characteristic appearance, being broadly oval with a stout albuminous coat, a rugose surface, and an inner vitelline membrane. When passed in the feces, they contain a large conspicuous ovum that, after being deposited in the soil, develops into an infective embryo in 10 to 30 days. Human infection is acquired by ingesting these eggs, which hatch in the small intestine.

The liberated larvae penetrate the intestinal mucosa to enter blood and lymph vessels. Some are carried to the liver, but those which are going to survive reach the lungs in 4 to 16 days after infection, where they penetrate into the alveoli and then molt. They then migrate via the bronchi, trachea, and esophagus back to the small intestine, where they mature into adults and mate. Eggs appear in the feces 6 to 8 weeks after infection.

Pathology

During the migratory phase, many of the larvae die, and these may induce a hypersensitivity reaction. Passage through the lungs may be accompanied by cellular infiltration, edema, and small hemorrhages. The adult worms, living freely in the lumen of the small bowel, feeding on intestinal contents, do little harm. In heavily infected children, however, hundreds of worms can form an entangled bolus, causing intestinal obstruction, which may be further complicated by perforation. Volvulus and intussusception have also been described.

Clinical Features

Passage of the worms through the lungs may be accompanied by low fever, some dyspnea, wheezing, and urticaria; occasionally these symptoms may be severe enough to cause the "ascarid pneumonia" syndrome. This is characterized by fever, paroxysmal cough with mucoid or blood-tinged sputum, substernal discomfort, breathlessness, and wheezing. Larvae may be found in the sputum. The chest X-ray may reveal discrete, rounded or oval soft densities, which often become confluent in the perihilar area. Serial films frequently show dramatic changes in both the location and extent of these shadows. A high eosinophilia usually occurs. The episode clears spontaneously in 5 to 10 days.

Heavy *Ascaris* infection in children causes colic, nausea, vomiting, or diarrhea, and may also induce a degree of malnutrition in those on a marginal diet. Subacute obstruction is suggested by a short history of abdominal pain and mild abdominal distension; an abdominal mass may be felt. Acute obstruction is associated with fever, vomiting, severe abdominal distension, and rebound tenderness.

The appearance of worms in the vomitus or in the nostrils causes more psychological distress than physical significance. Invasion of the biliary tract by wandering worms may result in jaundice, cholangitis, or even hepatic abscess; in parts of India, 40% of biliary disease has been attributed to ascariasis. In Hong Kong, the two common causes of acute pancreatitis are obstructions due either to *Clonorchis sinensis* or *Ascaris* worms.

Diagnosis

The diagnosis of ascaris pneumonia must be on clinical grounds, the presence or absence of eggs in the stools being irrelevant. Established infections may usually be confirmed by finding eggs in the stools.

Occasionally, all the worms are males so that no eggs are produced, but these worms may sometimes be visualized in a barium study. Worms in the biliary tract are identified by ultrasonography and endoscopic retrograde cholangiopancreatography.

Treatment

As intestinal helminth infections in the tropics are usually multiple, broad-spectrum anthelminthic drugs—such as albendazole, mebendazole, levamisole, pyrantel pamoate, and nitazoxanide—have largely replaced piperazine in the therapy of ascariasis. Anthelminthic drugs are contraindicated during acute ascaris pneumonia because producing more dead larvae will only exacerbate the allergic reaction; severe symptoms may be relieved with steroids.

Subacute obstruction can often be relieved by gastric suction, intravenous (IV) fluids, atropine, liquid paraffin, and saline enemas. If this is unsuccessful, or if obstruction is acute, laparotomy is required. The obstruction is commonly in the lower ileum, and sometimes the bolus can be manipulated through the ileocecal valve without opening the intestine. If this fails, the bolus must be removed surgically, and intestinal resection may be required. Biliary and pancreatic obstruction by ascarids can sometimes be relieved by endoscopic extraction of the worms. Finally, it should be noted that ascarid worms are attracted to sites of intestinal surgery, where they can digest sutures. Tropical surgeons should eliminate the worms before proceeding on elective abdominal operations.

Trichuriasis

Trichuris trichiura, the whipworm, is another geohelminth transmitted in a similar manner to *Ascaris lumbricoides*. These infections are commonly acquired at the same time.

The Parasite

The anterior three-fifths of the worm, bearing the mouth, is slender and filariform, while the posterior two-fifths is bulky and fleshy, the handle of the whip. The adult worms, approximately 5 cm long, parasitize the large bowel, where the female worm lays 3,000 to 7,000 eggs daily. The eggs, when they appear in the feces are unsegmented, but after 11 to 30 days in the soil, a coiled infective larva develops, and human infection is acquired by ingesting these embryonated eggs. The eggs hatch in the small intestine where, adhering to the villi, they develop into adult male and female worms. When mature, the worms pass down the intestine and parasitize the cecum and the ascending colon. There is no pulmonary migration.

Pathology

On colonic biopsies, *Trichuris* are found partially embedded in the mucosa. They attach to the bowel wall by the anterior, thread-like portion. They feed on blood and liquefied mucosal cells. In heavy infections, the cecal mucosa becomes hyperemic, and erosions occur, which may slough and bleed. In massive infections, the whole colon is involved, and rectal prolapse is common.

Clinical Features

The great majority of *Trichuris* infections remain silent. Massive infections with as many as 1,000 worms occur in children. They develop a chronic, profuse, mucoid and blood-stained diarrhea, abdominal pain, tenesmus, and rectal prolapse. Accompanying these symptoms there may be anemia, finger clubbing, and growth retardation.

Diagnosis

The diagnosis is confirmed by finding the barrel-shaped eggs with mucus plugs at both ends. They are double-shelled, the outer being bile-stained; and they contain an unsegmented ovum. Adult worms may be seen adhering to the mucosa at colonoscopy. It is important to distinguish severe infections from other forms of dysentery, and to consider this infection as the underlying cause in a patient with rectal prolapse.

Treatment

Treatment is as for ascariasis.

Hookworm Disease

Dublin (1843) recognized minute worms adhering to the mucus of the small intestine of patients who had died from other causes, and it was Greisinger (1854) who identified them as the cause of Egyptian chlorosis. Ashford (1900) and Bentley (1902) recorded severe infection among plantation workers in Puerto Rico and Assam, respectively. It is now realized that hookworm infection is endemic throughout the hot, humid regions of the tropics, and that when dietary iron intake is inadequate, hookworm infection may cause a severe iron deficiency anemia.

The Parasite

The parasites are minute roundworms, 1 cm in length, which live in the upper part of the small intestine with their mouthparts engulfing villi from which they draw blood. The two common species that infect the human small intestine are *Ancylostoma duodenale* and *Necator americanus*. They are readily distinguished by their mouth parts, *A. duodenale* having two pairs of fixed teeth, and *N. americanus* two crescentic cutting plates.

The oval eggs, 40 to 80 micrometers in length, have a glassy clear or yellow appearance and a delicate outer wall, and contain 2 to 8 cells, according to their state of development. When passed in feces on warm, moist soil, rhabditiform larvae hatch within 1 to 2 days and then migrate down into the soil where they feed on bacteria. After several days of growth and molting, motile, nonfeeding, infective filariform larvae are formed, which rise to the surface, where they may remain viable for 1 to 3 months.

Human infection occurs when individuals walk barefoot or farm on contaminated ground. The larvae penetrate the skin and are carried by lymph and blood to the lungs where they begin an active migration similar to that of ascarid larvae. Eggs appear in the stools 5 or more weeks after infection. In addition to the percutaneous route, *A. duodenale* can infect by ingestion of contaminated food.

Infantile hookworm disease due to *A. duodenale* has been predominantly described from China. Transmission occurs by transmammary route, by laying infants on contaminated soil, or on diapers made up of a cloth bag stuffed with contaminated soil.

The clinical features include bloody diarrhea, melena, vomiting, and massive hemorrhage with a mortality of 12%.

Pathology

A skin lesion may occur at the site of penetration, and hypersensitivity and pulmonary symptoms may develop during migration of the larvae, but are usually of a minor nature. The adult worms may traumatize the intestinal mucosa, but the most important cause of disease is blood loss in heavy infections. Each *A. duodenale* removes 0.15 ml of blood daily and *N. americanus* 0.03 ml. Each milliliter of blood contains 0.5 mg of iron, but nearly one-half of this is reabsorbed. Given that worm loads exceeding 60,000 have been reported, the amount of iron lost may be considerable.

The degree of resulting anemia depends upon the number and species of worms, the duration of infection, the dietary iron intake, and the iron stores of the patient. Serum albumin is also lost, and although the amino acids are reabsorbed, this loss may exceed the liver's capacity for resynthesis.

Clinical Features

The cutaneous lesion at the site of penetration of the larvae is usually insignificant, but when exposure is severe, as when rains swamp heavily contaminated ground on which barefoot people are working, it may be severe. Under these circumstances, an extremely irritating, erythematous, edematous eruption develops, followed by vesiculation and often pustulation. Migration of the larvae through the lungs results in wheezing, a dry cough, fever, and a high eosinophilia. Four to 6 weeks later, there may be vague abdominal discomfort, loss of appetite, flatulence, or even nausea, vomiting, and diarrhea. These early symptoms subside spontaneously, and most of those infected suffer no further ill effects.

However, heavy infections in normal people—or, relatively light worm loads in people with compromised iron stores—may be followed by anemia of varying degree. As iron absorption rises in response to a fall in iron stores, the onset is usually very gradual. Patients complain of slowly increasing weakness, fatigue, palpitations, breathlessness, and an inability to carry on with their work. People with dark complexions develop a grayish hue. The mucous membranes become pale, the face puffy, and there may be edema due to hypoalbuminemia. The general state of nutrition may appear quite satisfactory, and nail changes are seldom seen. Those particularly at risk include young children; field workers (often women); and pregnant and lactating women, who often present with a desperately severe anemia and congestive heart failure (CHF).

When infection with *A. duodenale* occurs orally, the migrations of larvae result in a syndrome known as "Wakana disease," which consists of nausea, vomiting, pharyngeal irritation, cough, dyspnea, and hoarseness.

Diagnosis

Laboratory confirmation of hookworm infection is provided by finding the ova in the stools, but the diagnosis of hookworm disease requires an estimate of the number of these eggs. Such an estimate may be obtained by using the Kato technique, but for all practical purposes, an experienced technician is well able to distinguish a significant and heavy infection from a light and insignificant one. The eggs need to be distinguished from those of *Trichostrongylus spp.* and *Ternidens diminutus*. The former are much larger than hookworm eggs, but the latter can be distinguished only by hatching techniques and differentiation of larvae following egg culture.

In anemic patients, the laboratory findings are typical of iron deficiency anemia. The red blood cell (RBC) morphology is hypochromic and microcytic, the MCH and MCV being reduced in proportion to the degree of anemia. The bone marrow reveals normoblastic hyperplasia and complete absence of iron. The plasma iron and serum ferritin are reduced, and iron binding capacity is markedly increased.

Treatment

Among indigenous populations in the tropics where reinfection is almost inevitable, treatment is indicated only when there is evidence of hookworm disease, except in children and pregnant women. Albendazole, mebendazole, or nitazoxanide are the anthelminthics of choice. Tetrachlorethylene should be abandoned because of its toxic effects and because it stimulates migration of ascarids, which are commonly present. Tourists and patients who have left endemic areas with even light hookworm infections usually demand therapy, and because it is so safe and effective, physicians in temperate climates should prescribe albendazole or mebendazole.

Mild and moderate anemia is treated with ferrous sulphate, which should be given for 3 months after the hemoglobin has returned to normal. Severely anemic patients, in heart failure, require careful management, and emergency transfusion may be needed. This should be limited to 1 unit of packed red cells and covered, if necessary, by diuretics to avoid circulatory overload. In pregnant women, exchange transfusion, if available, may be life-saving. The increase in hemopoesis following treatment with iron may uncover an associated folate deficiency requiring treatment.

Strongyloidiasis

Strongyloides stercoralis was first recognized by Normand (1876) in the feces of French colonial soldiers who had been suffering from uncontrollable diarrhea in Cochin China. Because the mode of infection is similar to that of hookworms, both infections are commonly found in the same individual. Infection may persist for life irrespective of external reinfection.

The Parasite

The adult female worms, measuring 2.2 mm in length, are found toward the base of the duodenal and jejunal mucosal villi or in the submucosa. The males do not enter the intestinal mucosa and are passed in the feces. During a lifespan of at least 6 years, each female worm deposits several dozen eggs each day. Rhabditiform larvae hatch out *in situ* and make their way into the lumen of the intestine to be passed in the feces. In the warm, moist soil of the tropics, a persistent cycle of rhabditiform parasites develops, but some of the rhabditiform larvae metamorphose into long, delicate filariform infective larvae that may remain viable for several weeks.

Human infection occurs when these larvae penetrate the skin, usually of the feet, and a migration follows as with hookworms. Infection can persist because some of the rhabditiform larvae convert to infective filariform larvae while still in the lower bowel or on the perianal skin, resulting in autoinfection. If there is delay in the passage of filariform larvae up the bronchial tree, adult female worms may occasionally invade the respiratory mucosa. The autoinfection cycle appears to be at least partially controlled by an immune process.

Pathology

The arrival of the adult worms in the intestinal mucosa appears to result in mast cell stimulation and local edema as well as a high eosinophilia. Later, this reaction subsides, and although the worms continue to burrow through the mucosa and submucosa, they elicit little reaction.

Clinical Features

Ground itch, urticaria, and pulmonary symptoms associated with larval migration are usually mild. The arrival of the worms in the intestine may be associated with an acute malabsorption syndrome with steatorrhea but normal D-xylose absorption. The blood eosinophil count may exceed 25,000 per mm^3. The subsequent course of strongyloidiasis is usually silent although heavy infection may be associated with attacks of abdominal pain or colic. Rarely patients may present with respiratory symptoms, cough, and wheezing, as well as rhabditiform larvae in the sputum. Other chronically infected individuals suffer from recurrent episodes in which a linear, serpiginous, urticarial rash appears on the buttocks, groin, or trunk—larva currens—only to disappear after a few hours.

Diagnosis

The diagnosis may be confirmed by finding rhabditiform larvae in fecal smears. The excretion of larvae may be both sparse and variable; duodenal aspiration gives more reliable results. Alternatively, a stool specimen may be cultured at 86°F for a few days; the larvae must then be distinguished from those of hookworm. An immunofluorescent antibody test using filariform larvae of *Stercoralis ratti* is claimed to be sensitive and specific. A low eosinophilia commonly persists.

Treatment

Ivermectin in a singe dose of 200 per kg is the treatment of choice. Albendazole is an alternative treatment, but therapeutic failure does occur.

Disseminated Strongyloidiasis

The most serious manifestation of *Strongyloides stercoralis* infection occurs as a result of massive autoinfection. This appears to be associated with loss of partial immunity and is seen with malnutrition and pregnancy; in HIV/AIDS patients; or following treatment of leprosy, lymphoma, or leukemia with corticosteroids or cytotoxic drugs. It is a particular hazard of transplant treatment in patients who have persisting subclinical *Strongyloides* infection.

Massive penetration of the bowel by infective filariform larvae takes place, the larvae being distributed throughout the body, but particularly in the mesenteric lymph nodes, duodenal and jejunal mucosa, liver, and lungs. Segments of the upper small intestine become grossly thickened and edematous, and fecal organisms may be carried into the cerebrospinal fluid (CSF).

Clinical Features. The illness may start gradually as a form of subacute intestinal malabsorption, but in patients being treated with steroids or cytotoxic drugs, the onset is often acute. The most common presentation is with a severe protein-losing enteropathy in which there is profuse diarrhea, steatorrhea, hypokalemia, and hypoalbuminemia. Alternatively, patients may present with acute duodenal obstruction and severe vomiting. A barium study may reveal a "pipe stem" deformity, usually affecting the lower duodenum and upper jejunum; on endoscopy, a grossly thickened, turgid duodenal mucosa may be found causing almost total obstruction. In other patients, a hacking cough with white frothy sputum may rapidly progress to severe dyspnea, with or without hemoptysis, and sudden respiratory failure. Chest x-ray reveals bilateral shadowing similar to the appearance of acute pulmonary edema. Still other patients present with an acute meningitis due to *Escherichia coli*, a passenger bacteria attached to the disseminating strongyloides larvae.

Diagnosis. After the diagnosis is considered, it is easily confirmed as the feces, duodenal aspirates, and sometimes the sputum swarm with larvae. If there has been a previous eosinophilia, this will probably have disappeared; the lower the eosinophil count, the worse the prognosis.

Treatment. Emergency treatment of the enteropathy, respiratory failure, or meningitis is required. The infection will usually respond to ivermectin given in the usual dose for 10 days. The drug may have to be delivered as a suspension through a duodenal tube. Further courses of ivermectin or albendazole should be given monthly for 6 months.

It is important that any patient who has been exposed to *Strongyloides* infection, even many years previously, and is about to begin steroid or cytotoxic drug therapy, should be protected against this catastrophic illness. There may be no history of proved diagnosis, no eosinophilia, and larvae may not be found in the stools, but such patients should be given 1 dose of ivermectin or a 3-day course of thiabendazole. If evidence of *Strongyloides* infection is present, a 10-day course should be given.

Prevention of Geohelminth Infections

The widespread contamination of the warm, moist soil of many tropical regions by indiscriminate defecation and the use of untreated night soil as a fertilizer ensures ideal conditions for the dissemination and survival of the embryonated eggs or larvae of these worms. The eggs of *A. lumbricoides* and *T. trichiura* are conveyed to the mouths of children on contaminated hands. Bare feet offer no protection against hookworms or *Strongyloides* infection. Effective single dose therapy is available. It has now been shown that mass chemotherapy will reduce clinical disease even though it does not interrupt the transmission cycle. Although reinfection is likely—unless environmental sanitation is simultaneously improved—the short-term relief from the burden of geohelminth infections is considered a cost-effective intervention.

The World Health Assembly has urged countries to control soil-transmitted helminthiases. The global target is to provide treatment to 75% of all school-age children, as well as many preschool children and pregnant women as possible. Mebendazole and albendazole are now available generically at very low cost.

Other Intestinal Nematodes

Other nematodes infecting the human intestine in the tropics include *Enterobius vermicularis*, *Trichostrongylus spp.*, and *Ternidens diminuta*. *Strongyloides fulleborni*, a relatively common parasite of chimpanzees and African baboons, may infect man, and the closely related *Strongyloides fulleborni kellyi* causes a "swollen baby" syndrome with general edema, abdominal distension, and respiratory distress in infants in

Papua New Guinea. *Capillaria philippinensis* is another worm that invades the small intestinal mucosa. Infection is acquired by eating raw freshwater fish, and results in a severe protein-losing enteropathy with malabsorption rather similar to that seen with massive *Strongyloides* autoinfection. *Capillaria* eggs resemble those of *T. trichiura*. Infection with this worm has been reported from the Philippines, Thailand, Iran, and Egypt.

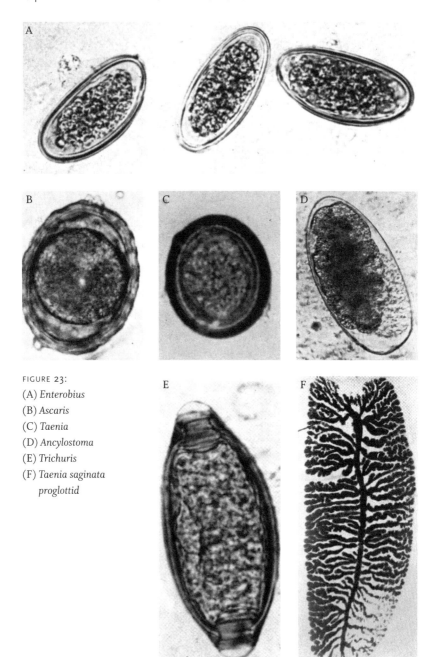

FIGURE 23:
(A) *Enterobius*
(B) *Ascaris*
(C) *Taenia*
(D) *Ancylostoma*
(E) *Trichuris*
(F) *Taenia saginata*
    proglottid

Intestinal Cestode Infections

These worms, although varying in size from 10 mm to 20 meters, have certain characteristics in common. They are flattened and ribbon-shaped. A minute head (scolex) attaches firmly to the intestinal mucosa by means of suckers, hooklets, or suctorial grooves. A short neck leads to a body made up of 100 to 4,000 segments (proglottids).

Nutrients are obtained by diffusion through the body wall; there is no intestinal canal. The worms are hermaphrodites, each proglottid having a complete set of male and female organs. The proglottids of different species may be distinguished by their shape and the appearance of the uterus. The eggs contain an embryo with six hooklets (hexacanth embryo or oncosphere). All species except *Hymenolepis nana* require a secondary intermediate host in which the larvae develop in a cystoid structure, usually in muscle. Human infection is usually acquired by ingesting raw or undercooked meat or fish. Drug treatment is with praziquantel.

Taenia saginata

The beef tapeworm may grow to a length of 12 to 20 meters, the body being composed of 1,000 to 2,000 elongated segments. The head is attached to the jejunal mucosa by four suckers, and the uterus has more than 13 lateral branches. The eggs, which are usually excreted within intact gravid segments, are spherical and have a thick wall that is radially striated. The intermediate hosts are cattle, which ingest the eggs deposited on grazing land.

Human infection is acquired by eating raw or undercooked beef or beef products, and also following contamination of hands while preparing raw meat in the kitchen. The diagnosis is confirmed by pressing a proglottid between two glass slides, and counting the lateral segments.

Although this long tapeworm, which may stretch from the jejunum to the rectum, seldom causes serious symptoms, the passing of segments and the wriggling of gravid proglottids through the anus causes distress. Infection is not regarded with equanimity by the almost universally infected cattle herdsmen of the Rift Valley of Kenya, and infected cattle are a cause of serious economic loss.

Taenia solium

This tapeworm closely resembles *T. saginata*. Its main importance is that both adult and larval forms parasitize man. Cysticercosis, the larval infection, will be discussed in the next chapter. The head of the adult worm is armed with two rows of hooklets in addition to the four suckers, and the uterus has less than 12 lateral branches. The eggs of beef tapeworms and those of pork tapeworms are indistinguishable. Domestic pigs are usually the intermediate hosts, but dogs are sometimes infected, and in areas such as southeast Asia where canine meat is eaten by humans, dogs play a significant secondary role in transmission. The fear of regurgitation of ova after treatment with the consequent development of cysticercosis is largely unfounded.

Hymenolepis nana

Hymenolepis nana, the dwarf tapeworm, measures only 25 to 40 mm in length. The head is equipped with four suckers, and a single row of hooklets mounted on a retractile rostellum. The body is composed of 100 to 200 squat segments. Infection is widespread in mice and is usually transmitted to man through the ingestion of food contaminated with mice feces.

A cysticercoid larva develops in the human intestinal mucosa, matures in 10 to 12 days, and then the adult worm breaks into the lumen of the intestine to attach to the ileal mucosa. Characteristic oval eggs, with a double membrane between which four to eight filaments arising from the poles may be seen, are passed in the feces. No intermediate host is required, and autoinfection is frequent.

Most infections remain silent, but heavy worm loads in children may cause abdominal pain, diarrhea, vomiting, and pruritus ani. The treatment of choice is praziquantel, which causes destruction of both worms and larvae. Endemic regions include the Mediterranean, Egypt, Sudan, India, and Latin America.

Hymenolepis diminuta is another very similar tapeworm of rats and mice, but differs from *H. nana* in requiring fleas, beetles, or other insects as intermediate hosts. Human infection occurs when children swallow these insects in grain.

Diphyllobothrium latum

Diphyllobothrium latum, the fish tapeworm measuring up to 10 meters in length, is also widespread along certain river systems in the tropics. The head is spatulate and equipped with two suctorial grooves (bothria). The proglottids, of which there may be 4,000, are short and squat with the uterus appearing as a brown, rosette-shaped patch in the center. The eggs, which are oval, operculated, and unembryonated when passed in the feces, are evacuated from pores on the sides of the segments.

If the eggs reach water, a ciliated embryo develops; and if ingested by a *Cyclops*, it will develop into a procercoid larva. When the *Cyclops* is eaten by a freshwater fish, the larva migrates into the musculature to develop into a plerocercoid larva (sparganum). Human infection occurs through eating raw or undercooked fish. Other definitive hosts include dogs, cats, and foxes.

These worms seldom cause symptoms. Although vitamin B12 deficiency may result from *D. latum* infection, this etiology is rare in the tropics. Of more clinical importance are other *Diphyllobothrium* worms, now known as spirometra, which cause sparganosis.

Intestinal Trematode Infections

Food-borne trematode infections affect more than 40 million people worldwide, with a high prevalence in southeast Asia and the Far East. The intestinal trematodes (flukes) are flat, leaf-shaped hermaphroditic worms equipped with a ventral sucker by which they attach to the human intestinal mucosa. If eggs, passed in the feces, reach fresh water, a miracidium is released and can enter and multiply in appropriate snails. Here, the parasite develops for several weeks into a cercarial form, and these are discharged back into water and develop further as metacercariae in or on a second intermediate host. This complex cycle is completed when man or a susceptible animal ingests the intermediate host. Treatment is with praziquantel.

Fasciolopsis buski

Fasciolopsis buski, the giant intestinal fluke of man and pigs, is a large, fleshy, oval fluke measuring up to 7.5 cm in length. The first intermediate hosts are Planorbid and other fresh water snails, and the metacercariae encyst on aquatic plants, such as water chestnuts, bamboo shoots, hyacinth, lotus, and calthrop. Children are infected when eating these plants or peeling them with their teeth; pigs are the reservoir of infection, which is endemic from India and Indonesia to China. Most infections remain silent, but heavy worm loads may cause abdominal pain, anorexia, nausea, vomiting, diarrhea, and loss of weight as well as an unexplained edema. The diagnosis is confirmed by finding the very large (130 to 140 micrometers) operculated eggs in the stools.

Metagonimus yokogawi and Heterophyes heterophyes

In contrast to *F. buski*, these flukes are minute, measuring only up to 1 mm in length. They are seen as reddish dots in the intervillous spaces of the small intestine, but may also penetrate the mucosa to cause a granulomatous reaction. The metacercariae encyst in the muscle of fresh water fish, and infection in man, dogs, cats, foxes, and other flesh-eating mammals occurs when raw or undercooked fish are ingested. Heavy worm loads may cause gastrointestinal symptoms. The diagnosis is confirmed by finding the small, red/brown eggs in the stools. Although these infections occur mainly in the Orient, *H. heterophyes* is also endemic in Egypt.

Larval Helminth Infections

Human disease may be caused by infection with the larval stage of intestinal helminthic parasites of animals. In the case of *Trichinella spiralis*, both adults and larvae are present, but in cysticercosis and hydatid disease, only the larval forms develop in human tissues. It need hardly be noted that only in exceptional circumstances does man become a true intermediate host.

Trichinosis

As the parasites do not exist outside mammalian carnivore hosts, infection is independent of climatic conditions, and trichinosis occurs in arctic, temperate, and tropical climes.

The Parasite

Trichinella spiralis is a small, slender nematode. The adult worms measure 1.5 to 3 mm in length. They live in the small intestinal mucosa and submucosa where, during a life span of 4 to 16 weeks, the female produces 1,500 larvae. The larvae, 100 microns in length, are carried by lymph or blood to all parts of the body. Those that reach transversely striated muscle penetrate into the cells where they coil up, and within 17 to 20 days, become encysted. In this situation, they may remain viable and infective for many years. After death of the larvae, cysts often become calcified. The life cycle is completed when a carnivore eats the flesh of an infected animal, and the cysts are digested by gastric juices, releasing infective larvae.

Pathology

Adult worms do traumatize the small intestinal mucosa, but the principal pathological effects follow the arrival of larvae in muscle cells. They elicit an inflammatory response with edema, swelling, cellular infiltration, eosinophilia, and a rise in serum creatinine phosphokinase. The myositis may persist for 5 to 6 weeks and then gradually subsides with encapsulation of the parasites. Affected muscles include those of the extremities, the diaphragm, intercostal muscles, the tongue, and eyes. Larvae may also be deposited in other tissues, such as the brain and the heart, where although they do not survive, they may cause a transient inflammatory reaction.

Clinical Features

Most infections are mild and pass unnoticed. More severe infections tend to occur in local outbreaks, such as when a bear is killed in Thailand, and villagers feast on undercooked meat, or following the killing of a bush pig or wart hog in Africa or a pork barbecue in Hong Kong. Heavy infections may be accompanied by nausea, vomiting, abdominal pain, diarrhea, or occasionally constipation. The main symptoms commence 1 week or more after exposure with a high fever, headache, myalgic pains, and severe malaise. Other features may include pain, tenderness and weakness of muscles, periorbital edema, and splinter hemorrhages under the nails. Blurring of vision, paresis, psychotic disturbance, cardiac arrhythmias, coma, and sudden death can occur. After 5 to 6 weeks, symptoms tend to abate gradually, but convalescence may be attended by persistent muscle pain.

Diagnosis

The diagnosis is suggested by the clinical picture, a history of recent ingestion of undercooked or raw pork, bear or bush pig meat, a high blood eosinophilia, and a raised serum creatinine phosphokinase. The diagnosis is confirmed by ELISA demonstration of specific IgE and IgM antibodies; muscle biopsy is seldom required.

Treatment

Severe symptoms are best controlled first by prednisone, 40 to 60 mg daily, and then specific therapy with mebendazole, in a dosage of 20 mg per kg bw for 10 to 30 days, to destroy the parasites. Mebendazole

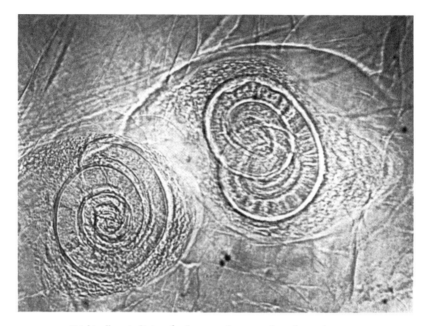

FIGURE 24: *Trichinella spiralis* in a fresh-pressed preparation of muscle.

is not advised during the first 3 months of pregnancy; thiabendazole may be used instead.

Cysticercosis

Man may act as host for the larval stage of *Taenia solium* as well as for the adult worm. This is most likely to occur where there is widespread contamination of the ground by human feces from individuals infected by the pig tapeworm. The most important endemic regions are India, South Africa, and Latin America. Outbreaks can occur among the most unusual contacts, as when a foreign domestic worker infected an orthodox Jewish Community in New York.

Pathology

The outer covering of the *Taenia solium* egg dissolves in the stomach, and the oncosphere is released in the duodenum. Here, it penetrates the mucosa and is carried by the blood stream to practically every part of the body. In the tissues, oval or round cysts develop over a period of 2 to 3 months, each containing an invaginated scolex with a crown of hooklets and four suckers. Except in the brain and the eye, a surrounding capsule forms from the host tissue reaction.

Human disease is largely associated with cysticerci in the central nervous system (CNS). In most cases, it is the death of the parasite that initiates a significant inflammatory reaction, accounting for the years that usually elapse before the onset of symptoms. The destruction of living cysts also explains the acute reaction that can follow specific anthelminthic hemotherapy. It is now clear, however, that cerebral edema, with or without seizures, may also be caused by the mere presence of young live parasites. Brain cysts are usually several in number, measuring a few millimeters to a centimeter in size. While viable, they are surrounded by a varying degree of local edema. Ependymal cysts may cause hydrocephalus by ductal obstruction. Occasionally, much larger cysts form, usually in the subarachnoid, and these may be racemose.

Clinical Features

The period between infection and the onset of symptoms varies from 5 months to 30 years, and most patients present with initial symptoms during the third or fourth decades of life. They most frequently develop severe, persistent headache, epilepsy, or evidence of cerebral hypertension. The type of epilepsy is variable, depending on the sites of the cysticerci. Cerebral hypertension may be due to cerebral edema or hydrocephalus, and is manifested by headache, vomiting, and papilledema. Less-common signs of cysticercosis are local neurological defects, extraocular palsies, abnormal behavior, dementia, or chronic aseptic meningitis. Subcutaneous cysts occur in up to one-quarter of patients. Unilateral loss of vision may be caused by a cysticercus in the eye, which appears as a white mobile cyst in the vitreous attached by a pedicle to the retina.

Diagnosis

A careful search should be made for any subcutaneous cysts, which after removal, appear as fluid-filled opaque bladders, each containing a

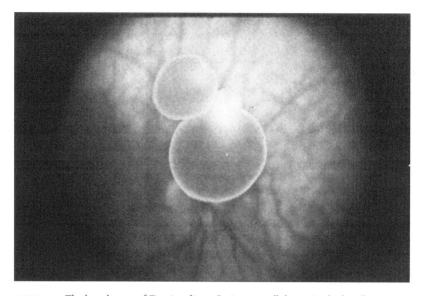

FIGURE 25: The larval stage of *Taenia solium*, *Cysticercus cellulosa*, attached to the optic nerve of a Guatemalan girl.

scolex. An x-ray of the musculature may reveal multiple, elliptical, calcified shadows. Affected cerebrospinal fluid contain eosinophils and an elevated protein concentration. Serological diagnosis has become more specific, using cysticercus fluid as the antigen in an ELISA test. The most helpful investigation, if it is available, is computerized tomography (CT). Viable cysts appear as hypodense images, sometimes including a hyperdense dot corresponding to the scolex. Following administration of contrast media, surrounding enhancement of the cysts, thus signifying edema, can be seen.

Treatment

Cysts outside the CNS or the eye are of little clinical importance. Symptomatic cerebral cysticercosis may be treated with praziquantel 50 mg per kg bw in 3 divided doses daily for 15 days. As the dying larvae may elicit a strong inflammatory response, this treatment must be accompanied by prednisone or dexamethazone, which should be started the day before, and only gradually tapered off following the course. This treatment, although highly effective, should not be embarked upon lightly; especially for patients with heavy parasite loads, high-grade neurological hospital facilities should be available. In many instances, control of seizures with anti-epileptic drugs is the only therapy required. Steroids are the first line of treatment for patients with cerebral edema although surgical decompression, especially for large single lesions, may still prove necessary. Albendazole is also an effective drug in a dose of 400 mg twice daily for 15 to 30 days; repeat courses may be necessary.

Hydatidosis

Alveolar hydatid disease is rarely reported from the tropics, but hydatidosis due to infection with the larval stage of the dog tapeworm, *Echinococcus granulosus*, is endemic in north Africa, the Middle East, and Latin America. The highest prevalence in the world is in the Turkana district of northern Kenya, where human infection rates reach 5% to 10% of the population.

The Parasite

The adult worm in the dog measures 3.6 mm in length, the scolex bears four suckers, and there are only three proglottids. The worms lie deeply within intestinal villi so that only the terminal segments are visible as chalky/white spots, an appearance referred to as "furring." The eggs, which can be distinguished from other tapeworm eggs only by specialized techniques, are ingested by herbivorous animals, such as sheep, goats, and camels. The onchospheres are mostly trapped in the capillary networks of the liver and lungs.

Hydatid cysts, which develop from single onchospheres, are composed of an external laminated layer lined by a nucleated germinal membrane from which fluid is secreted. Brood capsules, pedunculated vesicles containing scolices, develop from the germinal layer. As the pedicles break, they sink to the floor of the cyst and disintegrate. Daughter cysts arise from detachment of germinal nucleated cells; they resemble the parent cyst and may either float free or herniate through the capsule.

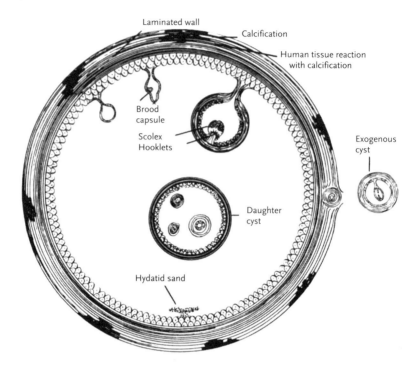

FIGURE 26: A diagrammatic drawing of a hydatid cyst.

Hydatid "sand" consists of scolices, hooklets, and calcareous particles derived from degenerated brood capsules. In most tissues, a fibrous capsule derived from the host forms around the cyst and tends to calcify following death of the cyst. Cysts grow at a rate of 1 to 5 cm every year and may reach the size of a child's head.

Pathology

Up to 80% of cysts occur in the liver and about 10% in the lungs. Other clinically important sites include the peritoneum, orbit, bone, brain, spleen, and heart. In these sites, cysts may be single or multiple. Pathological effects are due to the pressure of cysts on adjacent tissue, the leakage of fluid causing hypersensitivity reactions or seeding of new cysts, and secondary infection that can convert a cyst into a large abscess.

Clinical Features

Minor leakage of hydatid cyst fluid may lead to fever, pruritis, urticaria, and a rapid rise in blood eosinophilia. Major leakage, as after a motor car accident, may be followed by shock, dyspnea, and collapse. Rupture of a hepatic cyst into the biliary tree may be followed by biliary colic, urticaria, and jaundice. Liver cysts tend to remain asymptomatic and undetected for a long time. Their size, however, can cause upper abdominal discomfort, nausea, vomiting, and distension. A hydatid "thrill," a tremulous impulse over the cyst, may be elicited, and the diaphragm is often raised.

Pulmonary cysts are associated with a cough, productive of blood-stained sputum or clear "salty water." Posterior mediastinal cysts cause back pain and spinal erosion, while anterior mediastinal cysts may lead to tracheal compression. Orbital cysts cause painless proptosis, chemosis, and restriction of eye movement. Brain cysts usually present early with symptoms similar to those seen with cysticercosis. Cardiac cysts are a cause of sudden collapse and death. Bone cysts may be associated with considerable pain and tenderness, osteolytic x-ray appearances, spontaneous fracture, and neurological lesions from pressure on nerve roots or on the spinal cord. Splenic cysts usually cause no symptoms although they may grow to a very large size. A most distressing iatrogenic syndrome, following surgery, develops when a cyst leaks into the peritoneum, and the whole abdomen becomes tense and bloated with multiple cysts. In spite of all these possible contingencies, hydatid cysts are often a silent finding coming to light only in routine x-rays or at autopsy.

Diagnosis

The most precise and sensitive method for identifying hydatid cysts is ultrasonography. The rounded hollow lesions evoke echoes less numerous than those of amebic abscess, and weaker than those from tumor. Chest x-ray appearances are almost pathognomonic. Walled, roughly circular, cysts can be seen on fluoroscopy to change shape during respiration. A characteristic crescentic shadow may be caused by an airleak between the fibrous coat and the laminated layer. Alternatively, the

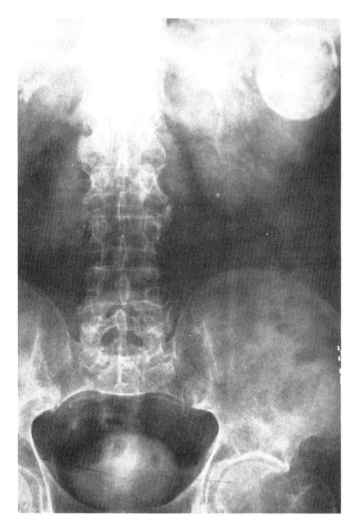

FIGURE 27: Solitary splenic cyst with characteristic calcific border and areas of increased density within the cyst structure.

laminated layer may collapse over a fluid level, producing the so-called "water lily" effect.

An elevated blood eosinophilia is found in only about one-quarter of those infected. Serology is notoriously unreliable. The old Casoni skin test has been largely abandoned, and most of the laboratory methods have either proved unsatisfactory because of cross reactions with other parasites or false-negative results. Recently, an antigen derived from immunoelectrophoresis of cyst fluid, the arc 5 antigen, has been developed. This gives a specific reaction with serum antibody using a double diffusion technique, but cross-reactions are common in patients with cysticercosis. Unfortunately, this test is not highly sensitive, and a negative result by no means precludes the diagnosis of hydatidosis.

Treatment

Treatment may be required if a cyst is causing significant symptoms or can be shown to be growing in size. The treatment of choice is surgical removal with special precautions during the operation to kill the scolices and prevent any leakage. Pulmonary cysts are removed by incising the capsule, followed by hyperinflating the lung, thereby allowing the cyst to be delivered intact. Surgical removal of liver cysts can be complicated by the spillage of cyst fluid or germinal membrane causing secondary abdominal cysts. This risk can be minimized by the prior injection of 1% centramide into the cyst, careful packing, the use of a cryogenic cone if available, and also the simultaneous administration of albendazole or praziquantel.

The previously intractable problem of dealing with multiple cysts and those not amenable to surgery has now been at least partially met by the use of albendazole. The principal metabolite, albendazole sulphoxide, reaches protoscopicidal concentrations in cysts and irreversibly damages the germinal epithelium. It is prescribed in a twice-daily dose of 400 mg with meals (10 mg per kg bw) for 28 days for 3 successive courses, each separated by 14 days. Cure is reported in 28.5% of cases, improvement in 51%, no change in 18%, deterioration in 2.4%, and recurrence in 13.8%. Liver function tests must be monitored throughout. Albendazole is also used before and after surgery and may be combined with praziquantel, which has an additive effect.

Epidemiology and Prevention

The epidemiology of hydatidosis is well illustrated in the hyperendemic region of Turkana. Here, the nomadic pastoralists tend herds of sheep, goats, and camels, 30% of which are infected with hydatid cysts. Each family has several dogs, 70% of which are infected with *Echinococcus granulosus* adult tapeworms. The dogs are fed raw offal. Because of the shortage of water, these dogs not only guard the huts but act as "nurse dogs," cleaning up the infants and young children. The soil floor of the huts, the surroundings, and the shallow water holes from which the nomads draw drinking water are all heavily contaminated with echinococcal eggs. It is, therefore, not surprising that "almost every lump turns out to be a hydatid, no matter in what part of the body it occurs." In many previously endemic regions, control of this infection has been achieved by the prohibition of feeding raw meat, especially offal, to dogs, by the treatment of infected dogs with praziquantel and the keeping of farm dogs outside human habitations. The chance of achieving control in Turkana, where water is at a premium, where there is little fuel to build a fire and where close contact of dog and man has become a way of life, seems remote.

Coenurus

Human infections with another polyembryonated larval stage of a dog tapeworm are reported from much of Africa. *Multiceps brauni*, like *M. multiceps* of Europe, is an intestinal parasite of dogs, with rodents as the usual intermediate hosts. In man, the coenuri present as subcutaneous cysts. The diagnosis is confirmed by the morphology of the parasite following surgical removal. Cysts may also be found in the brain and the eye, requiring surgical intervention and chemotherapy with praziquantel.

Human disease may also be caused by infection with helminthic larvae, which normally parasitize animals. In the abnormal human host, the parasites are unable to reach the necessary sites for development to maturity, and seem to wander through the tissues in an aimless fashion.

Cutaneous Larva Migrans

In the tropics, cutaneous larva migrans—or creeping eruption—is usually caused by the movement of feline or canine hookworm larvae in the skin. These parasites include *Ancylostoma braziliense*, *A. caninum*, and *A. ceylonicum*. As with other hookworms, human infection is acquired by infective larvae penetrating the skin. Larvae of *A. caninum* may occasionally reach the lungs and those of *A. ceylonicum* the intestine, but most parasites remain within the dermis.

The larvae move at a rate of up to 1 cm per day leaving a raised, red, intensely irritating, serpiginous track 2 to 3 mm wide. The intense itching leads to scratching, excoriation, and often secondary infection. This progress may continue for several days or weeks, but terminates spontaneously within 3 months when the larva or larvae die.

Treatment is either with a vanishing cream incorporating 10% thiabendazole or short courses of oral thiabendazole, albendazole, or ivermectin. Sandy beaches, sandpits, and areas under raised houses are likely sites for infection, and prevention lies in wearing protective clothing and by shielding suspect areas from animal fecal contamination.

Visceral Larva Migrans

Visceral larva migrans is probably more common in temperate regions than in the tropics. It is caused by infection with larvae of the dog roundworm, *Toxocara canis*. The eggs deposited on the ground in dog feces may be ingested by children, especially those afflicted by pica. The larvae migrate from the intestine, but are unable to find their way back and wander through the tissues and organs until they die. Death of the larvae initiates an eosinophilic granulomatous reaction.

Toddlers present with fever, nocturnal coughing with wheezing, hepatomegaly, and a high blood eosinophilia. Older children, adolescents, or young adults may present with unilateral loss of vision or a squint, and ophthalmoscopy reveals a lesion resembling a retinoblastoma. In these cases, there is no eosinophilia. The diagnosis may be confirmed by demonstrating specific antibodies. Treatment is with thiabendazole or diethylcarbamazine covered with steroids.

Gnathostomiasis

Gnathostoma spinigerum are small nematodes that live in tumor-like nodules in the stomach of cats, dogs, and many wild animals in southeast Asia. The female's eggs are passed in the stools and embryonate in water; the larvae, like those of *Diphyllobothrium latum*, mature first in freshwater *Cyclops* and then in freshwater fish. Frogs and poultry may also act as secondary hosts. Human infection occurs by eating certain traditional dishes, such as somfak, made with raw fish; or Labb kai, made with raw or undercooked chicken. Infection of the eye may follow the application of split-frog poultices, a traditional remedy for eye afflictions. The third stage larvae have heads covered with four to eight sharp, recurved hooks, and the anterior half of the bodies are covered with leaf-like spines so that during their wanderings through the body, they may cause considerable tissue damage.

The most common clinical manifestations are episodic, painless, pruritic, firm, nonpitting, cutaneous swellings of variable size. These erupt for 7 to 10 days and recur at 2 to 6 week intervals, which gradually increase, but episodic activity may continue for up to 10 years. Migration through the lungs may result in "pneumonitis" or pneumothorax; in the liver, right-upper-quadrant pain and low fever; in the urinary tract, hematuria; and in the uterine cervix, leukorrhea and profuse bleeding. Involvement of the eye is associated with pain, photophobia, lachrymation, periorbital edema, and subconjunctival hemorrhage. The most serious complication of gnathostomiasis occurs when a parasite enters the CNS. A sudden agonizing pain in the trunk and extremities is followed by severe, usually fatal, eosinophilic myeloencephalitis. Treatment is with albendazole.

Angiostrongyliasis

The adult parasite, *Angiostrongylus cantonensis*, a minute, transparent nematode, infects the pulmonary arterial system of rats. Larvae migrate through the respiratory tract and are eventually passed in rat feces. The intermediate hosts are snails, slugs, or flatworms. The life cycle is completed when a rat eats snails or other intermediate hosts. Human infection is acquired by eating the raw Pila snails of Thailand, the giant African snails of Taiwan, or the flatworms on fresh vegetables or fruit in the Pacific Islands.

In man, parasitic migration ends with the death of the parasites in the meninges, causing a self-limited eosinophilic meningitis. Severe headache, neck stiffness, but usually little or no fever, may be accompanied by a seventh nerve palsy and an intolerable, disagreeable skin sensation. A high eosinophilia is found in the cerebrospinal fluid. The condition resolves spontaneously, and anthelminthic treatment is contraindicated. Serum antibodies can be demonstrated after 10 days.

Angiostrongylus costaricensis

In Costa Rica, Brazil, and Mexico, another *Angiostrongylus* occurs as a parasite of the mesenteric arterial system of rats. The eggs lodge in the intestinal wall; the larvae migrate into the lumen and are excreted in the feces. The intermediate hosts are slugs, and children become infected when playing on the grass, their hands becoming contaminated with slug slime. Affected children develop an acute appendicitis-like illness with a high blood eosinophilia. Treatment is with thiabendazole.

Sparganosis

Spargana are the third stage larvae of the *Diphyllobothrium* tapeworms, *Spirometra mansoni* of southeast Asia and *Spirometra mansonoides* of the Americas. These larvae are creamy/white unsegmented, ribbon-like parasites, a few centimeters in length, each head bearing an invaginated slit. The life cycle of the tapeworms is similar to that of *Diphyllobothrium latum* although the second intermediate hosts are more commonly amphibians and snakes.

Human infection may occur by inadvertently swallowing infected *Cyclops* in fresh water; eating raw or undercooked snakes or frogs; or, as with gnathostomiasis, following the application of split-frog poultices to the eye. The most common clinical manifestations are migratory subcutaneous nodules. Eye involvement is marked by conjunctivitis, edema, retroorbital swelling, or corneal ulceration. Surgical removal of the worm or nodules is recommended. Although these plerocercoids cannot mature in man, an anomalous form, known as *Sparganum proliferans*, develops active budding with dissemination of the spargana throughout the body, a condition that may prove fatal.

Filariasis

Filarial worms are long thread-like nematodes that parasitize the tissues of humans and animals. In the tropics, they include some of the most important parasites of humans. Except for *Dracunculus medinensis*, the life cycles are very similar. The adult worms live in the body for 15 years or longer during which time, the female produces enormous numbers of immature, first-stage larvae, 200 to 300 micrometers in length, known as microfilariae.

The microfilariae do not develop further in the human body, but when taken up from the blood or skin by various arthropod vectors, develop into second- and third-stage larvae in the thoracic muscles of the insect host. The third-stage larvae enter the human body, completing the parasite life cycle, when the female arthropods take a blood feed. In the body, each infective larva may develop into a single male or female worm.

Wuchereria bancrofti Infection

Wuchereria bancrofti is the major cause of lymphatic filariasis, which is transmitted from man to man by *Culicine*, *Anopheline*, and *Aedes* mosquitoes in both urban and rural regions of the hot, moist tropics.

In 1877, Patrick Manson, working in Amoy, China, noticed that microfilariae began to appear in the blood of infected persons at about sunset, gradually increasing toward midnight, and then gradually clearing. He persuaded his gardener, who was infected, to sleep in a "mosquito house"; the next morning, he collected the blood gorged insects:

> I shall not easily forget the first mosquito I dissected. I tore off its abdomen and succeeded in expressing the blood contained in the stomach. Placing this under the microscope, I was gratified that, so

far from killing the filariae, the digestive juices of the stomach of the mosquito seemed to have stimulated them to fresh activity. And now, I saw a curious thing; the little sack or bag enclosing the filariae, which hitherto muzzled it and prevented it from penetrating the wall of the blood vessels in the human body, was broken and discarded.

In subsequent studies, Manson succeeded in tracing the filariae through the stomach wall, into the abdominal cavity of the mosquito, and then into the thoracic muscles. During this passage, the parasites increased enormously in size, developing a mouth, an alimentary tract, and other organs. This demonstration of transmission of parasites by arthropod vectors was to prove of fundamental importance in tropical medicine.

The Parasite

The female adult worm is a white thread-like nematode measuring 10 cm in length; the male is smaller at 4 cm. They lie coiled up in the lymphatic channels in a state of permanent copula, the female shedding microfilariae that reach the blood stream before they are extracted by mosquitoes. The rate of development in the thoracic muscles of the mosquito depends on temperature and humidity; at 79°F and a humidity <70%, it takes 12 days. The robust, sausage-shaped second stage larvae develop further into infective filariform organisms that escape from the mouth parts when the mosquito takes a blood meal.

They are deposited on the human skin, which they penetrate when the proboscis is withdrawn. They rapidly enter the subcutaneous lymphatics and are carried to the regional nodes. After a few days, the larvae migrate back down the lymphatic trunks; over the course of the next 3 to 6 months, they mature through two molts to become male and female worms. It should be noted that, as with all helminths, there is no multiplication of adults in the human body. Therefore, the severity of the illness can be roughly correlated with the number of worms initially injected.

Pathology

In most parasitic diseases, tissue damage is part of an immune response of the body to the infecting organism. Filariae, however, appear to be able to suppress host reactions, thus allowing for prolonged life in humans. In indigenous populations of endemic regions, where exposure begins in infancy and continues until death, the only evidence of infection in the majority of affected individuals is a silent microfilaremia. There is often no other indication of disease, and levels of serum antibody are minimal or absent.

In a minority of those infected, repeated attacks of lymphadenitis and lymphangitis occur, probably due to a host reaction to larval molting or from dead or dying adult worms. Endo and perilymphangitis affect afferent vessels and produce cellular hyperplasia in lymph nodes.

The lymphangitis is retrograde and is associated with endothelial cell proliferation, acute inflammation, and later fibrosis. Intermittent and, ultimately, permanent lymphatic obstruction occurs, the lymphatic channels becoming occluded and destroyed over considerable lengths; this process may be aggravated by secondary infection.

The obstructed lymphatics become tortuous, dilated, and varicose with incompetent valves, resulting in leakage of lymph into surrounding tissue spaces. This fluid has a high protein content and leads to a progressive disorder characterized by edema, chronic inflammation, and eventual fibrosis. The skin becomes thickened with deepened skin folds, hyperkeratoses, verrucae, and condylomatous changes. Abdominal lymphatics, and those draining the genitals, may also be affected; gross dilatation with saccular formation and rupture into the kidney or bladder can cause chyluria or lymphuria.

Clinical Features

Acute Lymphatic Filariasis

An acute onset of pain and tenderness in a single lymph node, or group of adjacent nodes, is accompanied by chills, fever, sweating, headache, weakness, and general aches and pains. Four to 8 hours later, an indurated, red streak may appear, running down the medial aspect of the leg. These symptoms increase over 24 hours, and then after 3 to 5 days, remit spontaneously, but similar episodes may recur at irregular intervals. Attacks are usually accompanied by transient swelling of the foot or ankle.

In some patients, an abscess may form in an inguinal or femoral node, burst to form a clean ulcer, and eventually heal by scarring; this sequence may be followed by freedom from further attacks. *Wuchereria bancrofti* has a special predilection for the lymphatics of the genitals; male patients can suffer acute attacks of orchitis, epididymitis, or funiculitis, and may develop a hydrocele. Rarely, patients present with acute peritonitis due to involvement of the abdominal lymphatics.

Chronic Elephantiasis

Chronic filariasis, the result of repeated infection over years, is due to permanent lymphatic obstruction. In lymphedema of the lower limbs from other causes, the swelling is usually nonpitting, and the skin is thin and shiny but of normal texture. In filarial elephantiasis, the initial stage is pitting edema; there is gross swelling, usually of one limb more than the other, with irregular bulging due to underlying fibrosis, bizarre skin hypertrophy, and nodular varicosities. The most common chronic manifestation of genital filariasis is a hydrocele, but elephantoid lymphedema of the scrotum or labia may occur. Obstruction and disorganization of the retroperitoneal lymphatics may lead to the formation of fistulae opening into the renal pelvis. These patients pass "milky urine," chyluria, or "pink urine" due to associated hematuria. Such attacks tend to be precipitated by a heavy meal but usually clear spontaneously. Persistent chyluria may lead to emaciation and edema. In a minority of patients, the arm or breast may also be swollen. Chylothorax is a rare complication.

Evidence has accumulated that secondary bacterial infection is a contributory factor in obstructive disease.

Acute Filariasis in Expatriates

When expatriates, or tourists in endemic regions, become infected for the first time in adult life, they commonly develop acute lymphadenitis and lymphangitis, but microfilariae are seldom detected in their blood. Of the 15,000 American servicemen infected during World War II in the Pacific, microfilaremia was detected in only 12. These men, after removal from the endemic zone, suffered no chronic effects.

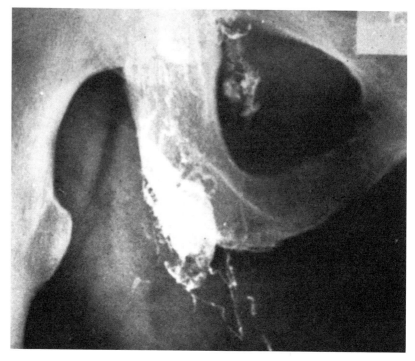

FIGURE 28: Filling defects in an inguinal lymph node, associated with the development of collateral lymph channels, in a patient with filarial elephantiasis of the leg.

Tropical Lung Eosinophilia

This condition is a hyperactive immune response to antigens released when microfilariae are killed in the lungs before they reach the peripheral blood. The mechanism of this destruction appears to be largely through activated eosinophils. The alveolitis, with subsequent granuloma formation and later fibrosis, appears to be due to a Loeffler-like hypereosinophilia syndrome.

Patients present with nocturnal cough, diffuse asthmatic wheezing with mucopurulent sputum, and a low fever. The spleen may be enlarged and diffuse lymphadenopathy occurs. The chest x-ray may be normal, but often shows striations or multiple hazy, patchy shadows, mainly at the bases. The sedimentation rate is usually elevated, but the most characteristic feature is an eosinophilia, which may reach 30,000 per mm³. Microfilariae are never found in the blood. Unless treated,

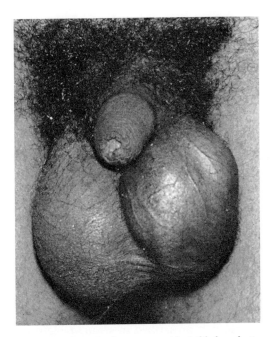

FIGURE 29: Scrotal enlargement with visible lymphatic dilation of the skin and hydrocele in a Haitian patient with filariasis.

pulmonary fibrosis with restrictive lung disease may follow. A variant of this form of filariasis is the Meyer-Kouwenaar syndrome, in which a massive eosinophilia is also associated with enlargement of lymph nodes, spleen, and liver.

Diagnosis

The diagnosis of *W. bancrofti* infection is usually confirmed by the demonstration of characteristic microfilariae in the blood. To avoid the inconvenience of having to take night blood, a dose of 2 mg per kg bw of diethylcarbamazine can be given, and the blood taken 45 minutes later. Thick films are stained with Giemsa or Field's stain. The microfilariae are sheathed and gracefully curved, and the tails are free of nuclei. A sparse microfilaremia is more easily demonstrated by passing 10 ml of hemolyzed or heparinized blood through a 5 micrometer pore filter.

Circulating filarial antigen can be detected with the use of mono-clonal antibodies using a dot ELISA technique, thus obviating the need of taking night blood samples. Commercial card tests are available.

Microfilaremia will seldom be demonstrated in patients with ele-phantiasis, nor in expatriate patients with acute filariasis, and never in patients with the tropical lung eosinophilia syndrome. Lymphatic fila-riasis is not the only cause of elephantiasis in the tropics. In parts of Africa, a similar condition is seen in people working barefoot on soil containing a high concentration of silica; the absorption of silica parti-cles through the skin leads to an obstructive lymphadenopathy pedoconiosis.

Treatment

Diethylcarbamazine citrate (DEC) is an effective microfilaricidal agent. It suppresses embryogenesis, and in full dosage, may lead to the death of the adult worms. It is prescribed in 50 mg tablets, each containing 25 mg of base. The conventional dosage is 3 to 6 mg per kg bw daily for 21 days; but in endemic areas, a single annual dose of 6 mg per kg. has resulted in a reduction of microfilarial density of 80% to 90% and is now the recommended regime. Moreover, it has also been shown that a single annual dose of 400 mg per kg of ivermectin is similarly very effective.

DEC may cause nausea and vomiting and should be taken after meals. Occasionally, more severe reactions occur, usually after the sec-ond dose, with fever, headache, prostration, and urticaria. Lymph-edema can be alleviated by regular washing of skin with soap and water, limb elevation, and topical application of antibiotics and antifungal cream. Surgical treatment of scrotal elephantiasis on the other hand is rewarding; it is almost always possible to save the testes and penis while removing redundant scrotal tissue. The tropical lung eosinophilia syndrome responds excellently to treatment with diethylcarbamazine.

Epidemiology and Prevention

This infection is endemic in certain parts of South America and Central America, the Caribbean, West Africa, and along the coastal regions of

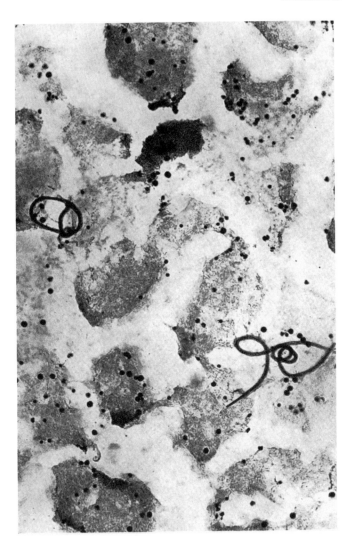

FIGURE 30: Thick blood smear with *W. bancrofti.*

east Africa. The highest prevalence is in India, southeast Asia, and the Pacific islands. Infection is common in the unsanitary slums of over-populated tropical cities, and in hot, humid coastal plains where holi-day resorts, complete with coral beaches and coconut palms, are concentrated. The reservoir of infection is the vast population of asymptomatic, microfilaremic individuals. The most important urban

vector is *Culex quinquefasciatus* (*C. pipiens fatigans*), which breeds prolifically in cess pits, latrines, domestic storage water, and drain pipes.
The common vectors in rural regions include *Anopheles gambiae*, *Anopheles funestus*, and *Aedes polynesiensis*. The mosquitoes are now largely
resistant to residual insecticides.

In China, India, and the Solomon Islands, diethylcarbamazine has
been added to table salt, resulting in a dramatic reduction of cases,
with microfilarial rates possibly falling below a critical point for transmission. It is ideal for this route because it is tasteless and stable upon
cooking, and has not led to parasite resistance. Vector control is also
required.

Because of widespread insecticide resistance, larvicidal measures are
of particular importance. The World Health Assembly has called "for
the elimination of lymphatic filariasis as a public health problem." Co-
administration of albendazole with diethylcarbamazine—and albendazole with ivermectin in African countries where DEC cannot be used
safely because of the concomitant presence of onchocerciasis—has
been shown to reduce significantly microfilaremia for a period of up to
2 years after a single administration. The free donations, for as long as
they are needed, of albendazole and ivermectin by drug manufacturers
have made it possible to put into effect the strategy of mass drug administration for the control of filariasis transmission.

Brugia malayi Infection

Brugia malayi is another important cause of lymphatic filariasis in
southern and southeast Asia and Indonesia. The pathological consequences of this infection are very similar to those in *W. bancrofti* infection except that the genital and abdominal lymphatics are usually
spared. The microfilariae have a kinked, rather than a graceful curving,
appearance and two discrete nuclei are seen at the tip of the tail. This
infection is more responsive to DEC than *W. bancrofti* infection, but
toxic side effects may be more severe so that a smaller dose is used in
treatment.

In contrast to Bancroftian filariasis, Brugian filariasis is largely confined to rural areas; there are two subspecies of the parasite. In Malaysia, one subspecies is nocturnally periodic, transmitted by both

Anopheline and *Mansonia* mosquitoes breeding in the rice fields and unforested swamps. The other subspecies, primarily an infection of monkeys, is confined to riverine forested areas. It is transmitted by *Mansonia* mosquitoes, and microfilaremia occurs in humans both day and night. Domestic animals may also be infected and serve as reservoir hosts. In Indonesia, one subspecies is transmitted only by *Anopheline* mosquitoes. Another separate species, *Brugia timori*, transmitted by *Anopheles barbirostris*, is now recognized on the islands of Timor and Flores. These microfilariae are longer, the sheath does not stain with Giemsa or Field's stain, and small terminal nuclei reach the tail. *Mansonia* mosquitoes obtain their oxygen from water plants, not from the water surface; control measures, therefore, focus on manually or mechanically removing these plants and by the use of herbicides rather than larvicides. The most practical method of community control, however, is mass chemotherapy with DEC and albendazole given once yearly, as for *W. bancrofti*.

Loaiasis

This filarial infection is limited to the great tropical rain forests and adjacent rubber plantations of Africa. The vector is the large red *Chrysops* fly of the forest canopy. Adult *Loa loa* worms wander through the connective tissue of the human body, and microfilariae appear in the blood mainly during the day. The adult female worm measures 5 to 7 cm in length, twice the length of the male. The cycle of infection is very similar to that of the other filarial worms.

Clinical Features

The bite of the *Chrysops* fly is painful, and swelling, itching, and redness may persist for a week. Several months later, the pathognomonic sign of loaiasis, the so called "Calabar swelling," may appear as a subcutaneous tumor 6 to 10 cm. across. It is usually preceded by local pain and pruritus. Common sites include the back of the hands, wrist, lower arm, or leg below the knee, but they may occur anywhere and may continue to recur at irregular intervals. They persist for a few hours to several days and then disappear. More disturbing are the migrations of adult worms traversing the conjunctiva, causing irritation, pain, edema, and lachrymation. Other less-common manifestations include temporary swelling of a whole limb, an abscess following the death of a worm, and an endophthalmitis that occurs after a *Loa loa* worm penetrates the eyeball.

Diagnosis

The diagnosis of loaiasis is usually based on epidemiologic evidence, classical symptoms, and a high eosinophilia. Microfilariae may be very difficult to demonstrate and are best seen at day time. The microfilariae, when found, are sheathed and kinked, and the nuclei extend into the tail.

A simple method using a questionnaire on the history of eye worm was shown to predict the level of endemicity of *Loa loa*. This rapid assessment procedure for *Loa loa* (RAPLOA) can identify communities which are at risk from ivermectin treatment.

Treatment

Diethylcarbamazine (5 mg per kg daily for 3 weeks divided into 3 doses) is the usual mode of therapy. Ivermectin 200 micrograms per kg is an effective alternative. Worms, especially in the eye, can be removed by surgery. Patients with a high microfilaremia ($>$3000 mf per ml) may develop an acute iatrogenic, potentially fatal, meningoencephalitis. These patients should first be treated with albendazole followed by DEC or ivermectin after the microfilariae count has been considerably reduced.

Epidemiology and Prevention

Chrysops silacea and *C. dimidiata* live in the canopy of the rain forest but descend to lay their eggs on plants growing in densely shaded, slow-moving or still, shallow water with a mud bottom. When the larvae hatch , they drop into the mud where they grow and molt for as long as 1 year. It is at this stage that the parasite is most vulnerable. Community control is best realized by clearing shade vegetation at breeding sites and by applying residual insecticides to the mud. Those at greatest risk from this infection are people living in small villages in the forest to which the flies are attracted by wood smoke. The flies will not enter houses unless they are well lit; therefore, screening is another form of protection. Personal prophylaxis with 300 mg of DEC once weekly has proven effective.

Onchocerciasis

Onchocerciasis is widespread in rural areas of tropical Africa and in Central America, South America, and Yemen. It is estimated that as many as 50 million people are infected. Although the great majority experience little inconvenience, along the rivers of the Sudan savannah zone, there are foci of heavy infection. Here, "river blindness" due to onchocerciasis, at one time affected as many as 50% of men older than age 40. In such areas, much of the limited fertile land had to be abandoned, and attempts at redeveloping these impoverished regions were doomed until this disease could be controlled. The Onchocerciasis Control Programme (OCP) has achieved this in the past 25 years, reducing transmission in 90% of the program area, treating 18,000 kilometers of river with temephos (Abate), and the mass use of ivermectin, resulting in the reclamation of fertile land and resettlement. In the whole OCP area (nine countries in west Africa), 200,000 persons have been prevented from going blind; 30 million have been protected from damaging ocular and skin lesions; and many millions of children now born are at no risk of blindness. A successful community control program.

The Parasite

Although the male adult worm of *Onchocerca volvulus* measures only 4 cm, the female may grow to a length of 70 cm. They tend to collect in subcutaneous nodules, where the female produces large numbers of microfilariae that invade the skin. The microfilaria do not develop further in the human body, and unless ingested by a feeding fly, die after 12 to 18 months.

Development in the thoracic muscles of the insect vector, the *Simulium* blackfly, takes 6 to 12 days. When an infected *Simulium* bites a person, the larvae implanted in the corium wander into the subcutaneous tissues. They do not multiply, but each survivor will grow into a single male or female worm that can survive for 15 to 20 years. Microfilariae appear in the skin 15 to 18 months after infection.

Pathology

In contrast to the other filarial infections, it is the microfilariae—not the developing or adult worms—that cause damage. Live microfilariae do no harm, but when they die, they become centers of inflammatory foci. This leads to a variable dermatitis and eventually degenerative changes. Microfilariae may also gain access to the eyes where their death may be followed by keratitis, iridocyclitis, choroidoretinitis, and optic atrophy.

Clinical Features

The earliest clinical symptom is intense itching over the lower back and buttocks. It may or may not be accompanied by a papular rash but is usually marked by excoriation due to scratching. In heavy infections, this stage is followed by a severe generalized dermatitis with gross hyperkeratoses, papules, and nodules. Loss of elastic tissue may result in a skin that resembles crushed paper, producing an aged appearance even in young persons. Another distinguishing feature is a patchy depigmentation, usually most marked on the shins. Subcutaneous nodules may be obvious but usually have to be sought; at first, they are firm and leathery, then later softer, and vary from pea to plum size. They are most frequently found behind the greater trochanters and sacrum in Africa, and atop the head in the Americas.

The death of microfilariae in the conjunctiva produces a gritty sensation associated with a brick-red conjunctivitis. Microfilariae can become entangled in corneal fibers, and as they die, cause "snowflake," "cracked ice," or fluffy opacities. This superficial keratitis does not interfere with vision and tends to remit spontaneously. Heavy repeated infections, however, lead to a severe, scelerosing keratitis with ingrowth of vessels and pannus, typically starting in the lower quadrants. These lesions gradually spread over the whole cornea, producing blindness.

Dying microfilariae in the iris may lead to a chronic torpid iridocyclitis with loss of the pigment frill. The iris texture comes to resemble yellow blotting paper or a pumice stone. The pupil is drawn downward, resembling an inverted pear. The development of posterior synechiae may lead to glaucoma and secondary cataract.

The first sign of retinal involvement is restriction of peripheral vision. Early funduscopic findings include small, pale dots and "cotton wool" areas. Later, one sees circumscribed zones of depigmentation that expose underlying sclerotic vessels with scattered collections of black retinal pigment. Optic atrophy is usual, the disc having a yellow/white appearance.

The manifestations of onchocerciasis varies in different regions. In the rain forest where infection is widely dispersed in time and space, where there is shelter from intense ultraviolet light and where the parasite may well be a different subspecies, most infections are light. Severe dermatitis, associated with inguinal lymphadenopathy, and edematous skin, the so-called "hanging groins," does occur, but severe eye involvement is uncommon. On the other hand, in the riverine areas of the savannah zone where the cycle of infection is constant and ultraviolet light is intense, eye lesions are disproportionately severe. An atypical form of onchocerciasis known as "sowda" occurs in Yemen and Sudan. The skin of one limb, usually a leg, becomes darkened, grossly thickened, and covered with papules and nodules. The lymph nodes draining the limb are enlarged, but microfilariae in the skin are very sparse.

Diagnosis

The diagnosis can usually be confirmed by finding the microfilariae in skin snips. The usual method is to raise the skin of the buttock on the point of a needle, and a shaving is then taken without shedding blood. The snip is placed on a slide or shallow dish of saline and examined under a dissecting microscope. Within a few minutes, agitation will be seen in the snip, followed by microfilariae wriggling and threshing out of the skin edge into the saline. Microfilariae may also be seen in the anterior chamber of the eye with an ophthalmoscope set at + 20 diopters. The efficacy of this examination is greatly enhanced by having the patient sit with his head between his knees for 10 minutes prior to ophthalmoscopy. A slit lamp, if available, makes the viewing of microfilariae easier. The Mazzotti test—giving 50 mg of diethylcarbamazine—can be used if onchocerciasis is strongly suspected yet skin snips are negative. Pruritus and a rash develop within 24 hours. The test should not be used if the eyes are affected. Specific ELISA tests and PCR tests are also available.

Treatment

Ivermectin, a macrocyclic lactone derived from *Streptomyces avermitilis*, given in a single dose of 150 mg per kg causes gradual destruction of microfilariae so that reactions, if they occur, are mild. It also temporarily inhibits embryogenesis and is now the standard treatment for onchocerciasis. It has no effect on adult worms. In areas where loaiasis and onchocerciasis coexist, ivermectin can cause a fatal encephalitis in patients with heavy *Loa loa* infection (>3,000 mf per ml). Because ivermectin is not macrofilaricidal, repeated doses at 6 monthly or yearly intervals may be required. Doxycycline has been shown to kill the endosymbiotic Wolbachia organisms in filarial species. Suramin is macrofilaricidal but is liable to cause severe toxic effects and has no action on microfilariae.

In Guatemala, where nodules containing the adult worms are found predominantly on the head and upper part of the body, nodulectomy is part of standard treatment. Severe blinding keratitis and secondary cataract are amenable to surgical treatment if advanced ophthalmic surgery facilities are available.

Epidemiology and Prevention

Onchocerciasis is transmitted by female *Simulium*, which are small black flies about a quarter of the size of a house fly. During the day, they are inconspicuous but may be seen crawling or hopping on bushes or grass in the vicinity of water. The black fly feeds in the early morning and evening, and its coarse mouth parts ensure that the bite is painful.

The vector in west Africa is *Simulium damnosum*; the female deposits eggs at the level or just below the surface of running water, often on rocks, stones, or any obstruction, such as the base of a bridge: that is, sites with sufficient water turbulence to provide oxygenation for the developing larvae and pupae. A special characteristic of this fly is its great range of flight; in a prevailing wind, it may be carried 100 miles. In east and central Africa, the vector *Simulium naevi* is found mainly in wooded upland areas; it has solved the problem of providing aerated water for larval development by laying its eggs on vegetation from which the larvae migrate on to the carapace of fresh water crabs. This fly has a much more limited range of flight. The African black fly bites mainly on the legs, whereas the Guatemalan vector, *Simulium ochraceum*, bites mainly on the upper part of the body.

Rapid epidemiological mapping and rapid epidemiological assessment of onchocerciasis, together with geographic information, systems are widely being used in endemic countries. The African Programme for Onchocerciasis Control (APOC), based on the efficacy, safety, and availability of ivermectin, is well established. The community directed treatment with ivermectin (CDTI) has proved successful and economical.

The only method of vector control has been spraying *Simulium* breeding sites, with Temephos as the preferred larvicide.

Other Filarial Infections

Mansonella streptocerca is a small filarial worm, measuring only 2.7 cm, and lives in the superficial tissue of the trunk and shoulder girdle. Microfilariae are found in the skin. The vectors are *Culicoides* midges of the tropical rain forests of west and central Africa. Dead microfilariae may induce a chronic irritating dermatitis on the upper trunk and shoulders. The microfilariae have to be distinguished from those of *Onchocerca volvulus*; they are shorter and have a sharply curved "shepherd's crook" tail. The microfilariae of other, nonpathogenic *Mansonella* also must be identified. Those of *M. ozzardi* may be found in the blood and skin snips of the inhabitants of South America and Central America. *M. perstans*, which infects as many as 50% of the population in forest regions of Africa, are found in the blood.

Dirofilaria immitis is a filarial worm that lives in the heart chambers of dogs (and sometimes cats) as well as the microfilariae circulate in the blood of these animals. Intermediate insect vectors include *Aedes* and *Mansonia* mosquitoes. Occasionally, the infection is transmitted to man. The parasites develop to near maturity in the human heart, but do not give rise to microfilariae. When a worm dies, it is carried into the pulmonary arterial system, where it becomes impacted and may cause a limited pulmonary infarction. In such a situation, a localized "coin lesion" can be seen on chest x-ray; on subsequent studies, it does not enlarge and eventually becomes calcified. The main danger to the patient is that the lesion may be misdiagnosed as a pulmonary carcinoma.

Dracontiasis

Dracontiasis is a disabling condition that once crippled as many as 40% of rural peasant populations at the very time when they were needed to plant or harvest crops. It is estimated that more than 3 million west African and Indian people were infected each year. It is a communicable disease that can be completely eliminated by the provision of safe drinking water.

The Parasite

The female *Dracunculus medinensis* grows to more than 1 meter in length, and when mature, its body is largely occupied by a uterus containing 3 million first-stage larvae. The larvae are discharged through the skin into water, following which the adult female dies. In the water, the larvae are ingested by fresh water *Cyclops* (water fleas), just visible to the naked eye. They develop in its body cavity into second- and third-stage larvae. When people drink infected water, the cyclops are digested in the stomach, and the liberated larvae penetrate the intestinal mucosa to reach the retroperitoneal tissues. There, they mature into adult male and female worms that mate. Following this, the male worm dies and is absorbed, but the female grows; over the next year, the female slowly migrates through the tissues to reach the skin, usually of the foot or around the ankle. The adult secretes a substance that produces a skin blister, which bursts to form a shallow ulcer through which the embryos are discharged during the next 4 to 6 weeks.

Clinical Features

Approximately 1 year after exposure, a localized burning pain develops, usually on the foot or lower leg. Simultaneously, there may be an acute systemic reaction with fever, urticaria, swelling of the face, dyspnea, or gastrointestinal disturbance. These generalized symptoms subside as soon as the blister bursts. The ulcer, surrounded by erythema and edema, remains intensely irritating, which encourages the patient to immerse it in cool water. Close inspection of the ulcer will reveal a minute hole in the center, which if douched, will after a few seconds produce a droplet of fluid, first clear and then milky, which flows over the surface. Sometimes a small, pellucid tube, the uterus, is seen projecting through the hole. If the milky fluid is examined under a microscope, it will be found to contain a myriad of embryos.

When the worm has successfully ejected its embryos, it gradually emerges from the ulcer that then heals, usually after 4 to 6 weeks. Unfortunately, before this occurs, secondary infection is a constant danger and may lead to cellulitis, which can prolong disability for months. Another danger is tetanus. Although about 90% of these lesions occur on the lower leg or foot, worms may be multiple and present anywhere. In India, water carriers bearing porous water skins on their back develop ulcers there.

Occasionally, worms may enter a knee joint and discharge larvae. This precipitates a sudden onset of fever, swelling, and tenderness, and the joint feels hot. Aspiration will yield a turbid fluid that may be mistaken for pus, but in fact contains larvae and no organisms. Other aberrant worms die and are visible as calcified shadows in routine x-ray films. Worms can also enter the vertebral canal, giving rise to an abscess with resulting paraplegia.

Treatment

The first aim of treatment is to reduce the size of the worm by encouraging the discharge of the embryos. The ulcer should be immersed in a bowl of clean, cold water for 30 minutes daily for 3 to 5 days. Alternatively, cold compresses with hypochlorite solution may be applied. When the worm is empty, it begins to extrude, and this process can be helped by winding the worm on to a stick or other rigid object. This must be done with great care so as not to rupture the worm, stopping whenever resistance is felt, leaving further extraction attempts for the next day. This process may take two weeks to complete. Meanwhile, the ulcer should be covered with a sterile dressing and antibiotic cream. Secondary infection requires systemic antibiotic treatment, and patients should also be immunized against tetanus.

Prevention

In endemic areas, water is still obtained from step wells, shallow ponds, or water holes into which people with infective ulcers must walk in order to fill their drinking utensils. Such sources of water can be modified by the provision of pump wells, tube wells, or draw wells, but a supply of safe piped water remains an urgent requirement. Meanwhile, control of *Cyclops* by the application of Abate or the introduction of *Cyclops* eating fish, combined with the boiling or filtration of drinking water, are effective preventative measures. Straining water through a cloth or gauze linen mesh prevents infection. The disease has largely been eliminated from Asia, and global disease eradication is a distinct possibility.

Schistosomiasis

In many parts of South America and the Caribbean, as well as throughout Africa, the Middle East, and the Orient, schistosomal infections are a clinical and an economic curse. It is estimated that more than 200 million people worldwide are infected: Most live in poor communities without access to safe drinking water and adequate sanitation.

Much of Africa is arid most of the year, and development depends on water conservation and irrigation from the great rivers. Many dams for the provision of energy and irrigation have been built in the past quarter century, but in nearly every instance, they have resulted in an increase in the incidence of schistosomiasis. Furthermore, a mild form of urinary infection is being replaced by the more severe intestinal disease. Infection is acquired by contact with still or slowly flowing fresh water contaminated by infected urine or feces. The most serious consequences occur in people living or working on irrigated land. Fortunately, new safe and extremely effective drugs are now available to not only relieve suffering but also prevent transmission.

The Parasite

Schistosomes are blood flukes 1 cm to 2 cm long that grow to maturity in about 6 to 8 weeks in the hepatic portal blood. The males have an elongate, leaf-like shape with the margins folded to form a groove, or "schist," in which the slender females are carried. Following fertilization of the female, both worms make their way against the blood current to the terminal vesicle or mesenteric plexuses. The female then migrates into, and obstructs, a small venous radical; here, it lays 300 to 3,000 embryonated eggs daily.

Over the next 8 to 12 days, these eggs, assisted by the secretion of a lytic substance and the contractions of the viscus, penetrate through the submucosa and mucosa into the lumen of the bladder or intestine and are shed in the urine or feces. If the eggs reach fresh water, the ciliated motile embryos, now known as miracidia, they must find and enter the tissues of an appropriate snail within 24 hours. During the next 4 to 8 weeks, massive multiplication takes place through sporocyst and redia stages, ending with the release of showers of cercariae into the water in response to light. The cercariae—the infective forms—are fork-tailed and just visible to the naked eye; they are highly motile, but cannot feed and must find a human or animal host within 48 hours to complete the life cycle. They enter the dermis, lose their tails, and become schistosomules. After 4 to 5 days, those that are going to survive are swept up by the circulatory system and ultimately reach the hepatic portal blood.

Pathology

There is little reaction to the intravascular adult worms. Pathological changes in schistosomiasis result from a granulomatous response to the presence of those eggs, which do not succeed in escaping to the bowel or bladder lumen. The embryo within the egg remains alive for about 4 weeks and steadily secretes a lytic material through the pores of the egg shell. This substance is highly antigenic, provoking a hypersensitivity reaction with the development of granulomatous inflammation. Some eggs are swept back in the venous circulation to a capillary plexus, where granulomatous reaction is also provoked.

The adult worms, although they do not multiply in the body, usually survive for 3 to 7 years but may live longer than 30 years. In endemic areas, the indigenous population is exposed to constant infection, and an enormous build-up of parasites can occur. Fortunately, this is usually prevented by the development of a partial immunity. Adult schistosomes produce antigens that stimulate host antibody as well as activate eosinophils that attach to and destroy invading schistosomules. The adult worms further protect themselves by incorporating host antigen into their tegmentum so that they are no longer recognized as foreign.

The natural history of all schistosomal infections can be conveniently described in three stages:

1. The stage of penetration
2. The stage of migration: "Katayama fever"
3. The stage of established disease, which at first is reversible, but if untreated, becomes irreversible

The stage of penetration by cercariae results in an itchy papular rash known as "swimmer's itch." The migration of schistosomules through the lungs gives rise to fever, malaise, urticaria, diarrhea, high blood eosinophilia, cough, and wheeze. The stage of established disease occurs when the adult worms reach their final habitat in the vesical plexus for *S. haematobium*, or the mesenteric veins for *S. mansoni* and *S. japonicum*, and eggs are released. Stages 1 and 2 (as described in the preceding list) are uncommonly recognized in children in endemic areas. Immigrants or visitors are the ones usually affected.

Schistosoma haematobium

Urinary schistosomiasis was first described in a Cairo morgue in 1852 by Theodor Bilharz. The disease, commonly called "Bilharzia" in endemic zones, is caused by *Schistosoma haematobium* and affects more than 100 million people in Africa and the Middle East. The intermediate hosts are aquatic, sinestral, turreted *Bulinus* snails, which breed prolifically in any still or slowly moving fresh water.

Pathology

The retained eggs in the bladder wall and ureters provoke a chronic cystitis and ureteritis. Large aggregations of endothelial cells, giant cells, and lymphocytes form; later, the wall fibroses, and the eggs calcify. Early lesions appear as tubercles in the bladder mucosa, often in the trigone area. Later macroscopic lesions include focal mucosal roughening, brownish staining, sandy patches, small sessile polyps, and sometimes superficial ulceration. The distribution of these lesions is usually focal and irregular. Strictures may develop in the lower ureters, and these can produce hydroureter and hydronephrosis. Secondary infection often occurs, causing stones to form in the renal pelvis. As the eggs die and calcify, the bladder becomes rigid. After a dozen years or more, metaplasia of the mucosal cells leads to a squamous carcinoma. Eggs may also be deposited in the rectal mucosa, the walls of the appendix and caecum, and the uterine cervix or vagina; rarely, eggs are carried back to the pulmonary arterial system to cause an obliterative endarteritis. *Salmonella* may also colonize the tegmentum of the adult worms leading to a prolonged bacteremia.

Clinical Features

The first symptom is usually painless, terminal, intermittent hematuria. In some regions, nearly all children are affected by the time they reach the age of 10; this is so accepted as part of the growing-up process that in young boys, it is considered analogous to the onset of menstruation in girls. Other less-common symptoms include a dull ache in the urethral or suprapubic areas before and during micturition, or a burning at the tip of the penis.

There are usually no abnormal physical findings. Nevertheless, even in asymptomatic patients, the urine contains protein as well as red and (often) pus cells, and examination of the blood may reveal a low eosinophilia. A plain x-ray of the lower abdomen may reveal calcification in the bladder wall. Pyelography or ultrasonography will often demonstrate polyps in the bladder and also ureteric obstruction with dilatation of the ureter and renal pelvis. Kidney function is usually unaffected in early cases. In the majority of those infected in childhood, signs and symptoms tend to remit spontaneously after adolescence or with treatment, but persisting structural changes may lead to problems in adult life. A significant minority pose difficult diagnostic challenges.

Some present with what appears to be an acute appendicitis. Laparotomy will reveal reddening and edema of the appendix and caecum with subserosal tubercles around *S. haematobium* eggs. Involvement of the uterine cervix may cause erosions and bleeding. Massive egg embolism can result in severe pulmonary hypertension and right-sided heart failure. A syndrome of chronic indolent fever, malaise, weight loss, and a petechial rash on the legs is seen in secondary *Salmonella* bacteremia. In regions where *S. hematobium* is endemic, there is a far higher incidence of carcinoma of the bladder, and they are squamous epitheliomas rather than the typical transitional cell neoplasma, and occur in middle age rather than old age. Involvement of prostate, seminal vesicles, and spermatic chord has been reported as well as eggs found in semen.

Diagnosis

The diagnosis of *S. haematobium* infection seldom presents difficulty. A specimen of urine, optimally obtained between noon and 2 p.m., is held in a conical glass for 30 minutes; the sediment is then aspirated and examined under a microscope for terminally spined eggs. Live eggs are clear and reveal a flickering embryo (flame cells). Alternatively, 5 ml of cooled, freshly boiled water may be added to the sediment, shaken thoroughly, and then left under artificial light at 72°C for 30 minutes; hatched miracidia may then be seen with a hand lens against a dark background. Eggs may also be sought by rectal biopsy, but this is rarely required except in light infections among expatriates. In rural endemic areas, the presence of 30 mg per 100 ml of protein and a trace of blood in the urine is often used as an indication of infection requiring treatment. Renography is now widely used to detect lesions in the urinary tract. Cystoscopy may reveal "sandy patches" in the bladder mucosa or leukoplakia. Antigen detection and molecular techniques are also available.

In endemic areas, a history of hematuria correlates well with the diagnosis of urinary schistosomiasis. However, the sensitivity and positive predicted value of reported hematuria as an indication of heavy infection is lower in persons co-infected with HIV. The parasitological cure rate and reduction in egg intensity is not affected.

Treatment

The drug of choice is praziquantel (PZQ), an isoquinoline compound given in a single dose of 40 mg per kg bw after breakfast. Side effects include epigastric pain, nausea, vomiting, rash, headache, and fever; they are seldom severe. Cure, as assessed by an inability to demonstrate viable eggs in the urine 2 to 3 months after treatment, is reported in 80% to 95% of patients. Another effective drug (now uncommonly used), is metrifonate, given in a dose of 10 mg per kg bw on 3 occasions at biweekly intervals. Successful drug treatment is usually followed by

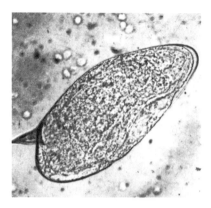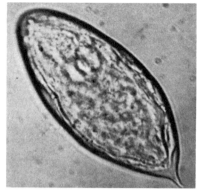

FIGURE 31: The lateral spined egg of *S. mansoni* (A) is found in the feces, while the terminal spined ova of *S. haematobium* (B) are seen in the urine.

considerable improvement in structural abnormalities of the bladder, ureters, and kidneys; surgical intervention is rarely required. Artemisinin derivatives can be used to treat acute (Stage 2) schistosomiasis.

Schistosoma mansoni

In contrast to *S. haematobium* infection, this form of schistosomiasis carries a significant mortality. The manifestations are varied, and clinical diagnosis may present considerable difficulty for inexperienced physicians. Although Bilharz (1852) and Greisinger (1854) both recognized the lateral spined eggs present in intestinal lesions, it was left to Manson in 1893 to suggest that these eggs came from a different species of schistosomes. This view was accepted by Sambon in 1907, who formally named the new species after Manson, "in appreciation of this, one of his many genial intuitions."

This infection is endemic not only in Africa and parts of the Middle East, but also in South America, especially Brazil, and in parts of the Caribbean. The intermediate hosts are aquatic, flat, *Biomphalaria* snails that breed in irrigation ditches and terminal canals.

Pathology

Schistosome eggs are deposited in the submucosa and mucosa of the colon and rectum near the inferior mesenteric venous plexus. Depending upon the intensity of infection, the eggs elicit a variable degree of colitis and proctitis, with localized areas of mucosal congestion, and erosion associated with a bloody, mucoid exudate. Along the Nile, polyp formation of the colon is common. However, in some patients with advanced *S. mansoni* infection, colonoscopic examination may appear to be perfectly normal, while biopsies reveal masses of eggs.

Eggs may be swept back in the portal blood to become entrapped in the liver, causing a granulomatous periphlebitis. The hepatocytes are not involved, and liver function is little affected, but presinusoidal portal hypertension is severe due to fibrous tissue surrounding the portal canals. The cut surface looks as if a number of white clay pipe stems had been thrust at various angles through the organ. This, in turn, may lead to massive splenomegaly and esophageal varices, rupture of which is a common cause of death.

Venous collaterals may also carry eggs into the pulmonary arterial system. leading to obliterative endarteritis, pulmonary hypertension, and right-sided heart failure. Immune complexes, normally removed by the liver, may be carried to the kidneys, causing a glomerular nephritis.

Proliferative granulomatous lesions also develop in the bowel wall, usually in the ileocecal region; occasionally, the entire peritoneum becomes studded, mimicking tuberculous peritonitis. Eggs may even be carried through the paravertebral plexus and deposited in the lower spinal cord. causing granulomatous inflammation.

Clinical Features

The clinical features of established infection vary widely. In many regions of Africa, routine stool examination will reveal *S. mansoni* eggs in apparently healthy individuals. In some localities, children may present with severe asthenia and hepatomegaly, and both will clear following treatment. In yet other areas, where the intensity of infection is presumably higher, children, especially, experience recurrent bloody diarrhea and hepatomegaly. In parts of Egypt and Sudan, colitis may be associated with pseudopapillomatous lesions of the lower colon and rectum, resulting in bloody diarrhea, finger clubbing, anemia, and hypoalbuminemia. Adult visitors to endemic regions seem to be particularly liable to an acute ulcerative colitis–like syndrome or to spinal cord involvement, the latter often being ushered in by acute urinary retention, followed by flaccid paralysis.

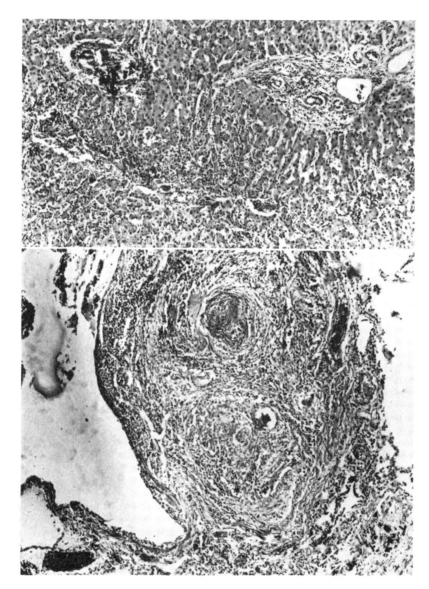

FIGURE 32: (A) Hepatic schistosomiasis with interlobular fibrosis, vascular dilation, and calcified ova. (B) Pseudotubercle formation in pulmonary schistosomiasis. Central calcified ovum, peripheral leukocytic infiltration, and granulomatious change are characteristic.

Hepatosplenic disease is usually only seen in individuals who have been exposed to heavy infection over a period of years. It has, however, also been described in persons who give no history of previous disease and who have lived outside endemic regions for many years. This syndrome usually presents with splenomegaly associated with anemia, leukopenia, and thrombocytopenia. Many patients are first admitted to hospital following severe hematemesis. The initial bleed is rarely fatal, liver function being well preserved, but subsequent hemorrhages often end with death. Since the widespread use of praziquantel, hepatosplenic disease due to S. mansoni has become quite uncommon in Egypt.

Patients with pulmonary hypertension and right-sided heart failure will complain of tiredness, syncope, and chest pain rather than breathlessness. They often have engorged jugular veins, tricuspid incompetence, clear lung fields with grossly enlarged pulmonary arteries, and severe right ventricular stress. The nephrotic syndrome with massive proteinuria, hypoalbuminemia, and generalized edema is another complication of hepatosplenic schistosomiasis.

Diagnosis

Observing viable, laterally spined eggs in the stools or in rectal or colonic biopsies confirms the diagnosis. Concentration techniques increase the chance of finding eggs. Histologic sections should be cut thick and examined under low-power microscopy, or alternatively, a fresh biopsy may be directly examined between two slides. A persistent low eosinophilia is a frequent clue in suspicious cases. Circumoval precipitation test is but one of several serologic tests that can be of use in difficult differential diagnoses. Antigen detection and molecular techniques are now available. Hepatosplenic disease may be confirmed by ultrasonography, revealing thickening of portal vein radicals and obliteration of the central translucency in peripheral hepatic vessels and portal fibrosis. Severe hepatosplenic disease may be present in patients with normal colon examinations.

Treatment

Praziquantel is the drug of choice; 40 mg per kg bw is given as a single oral dose. Treatment may be followed a few hours later by severe abdominal pain and the passage of several bloody stools. Reported cure rates vary from 60% to 90%. Another drug that is also effective is oxamniquine. Side effects include discolored urine, dizziness, drowsiness, and rarely, epileptic fits.

Patients with spinal cord lesions have been treated with praziquantel in a dose of 75 mg per kg bw given with corticosteroids. The treatment of hepatosplenic disease is unsatisfactory; surgical removal of a large spleen is an extremely hazardous procedure, especially in regions where blood for transfusion is either limited or liable to be infected. Esophageal varices may be treated by sclerotherapy, but portacaval shunts have given discouraging results. The nephrotic syndrome associated with chronic *Salmonella* infection responds well to antibiotic treatment.

Schistosoma japonicum

Schistosoma japonicum is the etiologic agent of Oriental schistosomiasis; it is endemic in China, the Philippines, and Indonesia. The intermediate hosts are small, conical, amphibious snails found in canals, irrigation ditches, and rice fields. In 1847, Daijiri Jujii wrote his *Katayama Memoirs*, an account of a journey to the southern tip of Honshu Island in Japan. During the spring and summer, farmers working in the flooded rice fields there developed irritating rashes on the legs, and some weeks later, an illness with heavy night sweats and bloody diarrhea. Other villagers displayed a drum-like distension of the abdomen associated with dilated abdominal veins and anasarca. The parasites, pathology, and clinical features of this infection closely resemble those seen in *S. mansoni* infection so that only differences will be cited.

The Parasite

The female lays 10 times more eggs than *S. mansoni*; these eggs are oval and smaller and have a minute lateral tubercle. Cats, dogs, cattle, and other animals are also infected; this is in contrast with *S. haematobium* and *S. mansoni*, in which animal reservoirs play no significant role in transmission.

Pathology

The pathological features are similar but may be more extensive, involving the lower small bowel in addition to the colon and rectum. Extensive hepatosplenic disease occurs, and expanding granulomatous lesions are found in the brain as well as the lower part of the spinal cord.

Clinical Features

In regions of intense transmission, cercarial dermatitis and the Katayama syndrome tend to be severe. Victims experience acute pulmonary symptoms, marked urticaria, and local edema. Dysentery may be prolonged and merges into the later stage of hepatosplenic disease. In some patients, the first serious manifestation may be due to a central nervous system granuloma, with epilepsy and/or evidence of an expanding intracranial mass. In the Philippines and Indonesia, where infection tends to be less intense, many infections are subclinical.

Diagnosis

The diagnosis is confirmed by the same parasitological and serologic techniques used for *Schistosoma mansoni*. Chinese field workers have developed a simple but very effective method. A fecal specimen, placed in a test tube, is covered with a ball of cotton wool and water. After 12 hours of incubation, actively motile miracidia may be seen swimming in the upper portion of the water.

Treatment

The only satisfactory drug for the treatment of this infection is praziquantel (60 mg per kg bw) given orally in 2 doses, 6 hours apart. The cure rate for a single course is reported as being 60% to 80%. Even cerebral lesions respond to treatment with praziquantel and corticosteroids; surgery is usually contraindicated.

Other Schistosomal Infections

Schistosoma intercalatum infects man in west and central Africa and in Sao Tome in the Gulf of Guinea. The clinical effects resemble mild

Mansoni schistosomiasis, but the eggs have a terminal spine that is usually slightly bent. *S. matthei*, a parasite of sheep, cattle, horses, and antelopes in South Africa, occasionally infects man. *S. mekongi* closely resembles *S. japonicum* and is endemic along the lower Mekong River. Treatment of all these infections with praziquantel is effective.

The Prevention and Control of Schistosomiasis

Control measures include reducing the number of miracidia shed into fresh water, destroying snails, and providing safe water to households. Until recently, success has been very limited, but now the availability of potent molluscicides and effective, safe, convenient therapy for all infected persons has revolutionized the outcome. Current control programs are based on

1. Mass or selective chemotherapy of the resident population with praziquantel, 40 mg per kg bw every 12 months for 2 years
2. Targeted chemotherapy with praziquantel 40 mg per kg bw to all school-age children in endemic areas at regular intervals, the frequency depending on the degree of transmission
3. Health education and the provision of adequate latrines, including communal, in-field, cemented toilet facilities in irrigation areas
4. Maintenance of free-flowing water by the removal of weeds and other obstructions from canals and irrigation ditches
5. Periodic focal molluscicide applications (based on man-water contact studies) either by steady drip feed of niclosamide into branch canals or by spraying of drains, irrigation ditches, and other major water contact points
6. Establishing villages at a safe distance from irrigation zones, and providing stored, piped water to each household and communal laundry
7. It has recently been shown that doses of artemether given every 3 weeks can prevent all three schistosomal infections. The value of this intervention is limited because of the logistics involved and current cost of the drug. Because artemether kills the schistosomules, a good indication for its use is in the expatriates

who give a history of exposure but in whom eggs have not yet appeared.

National control programs, using praziquantel at regular intervals, depending on the degree of endemicity, have reduced serious morbidity in Egypt, Brazil, and China. To date, more than 20 projects targeting 45 million school-age children are being supported in Africa. After minimal training, teachers—as are other respected individuals for community-directed mass treatment—are now able to distribute PZQ to school-age children.

Other Trematode Infections

Other trematodes, or flukes, cause significant human disease, especially in the Far East. The public health and economic impact of food-borne trematode infections is considerable in terms of morbidity, loss of productivity, health care costs, and agricultural loss. The adult parasites are flat, elongate, reddish/brown hermaphrodites, 1 to 2 cm in length. The eggs, which vary in size, are pitcher-shaped and operculated, and reach the exterior in the feces or sputum of the definitive host. On reaching fresh water, the eggs hatch and the miracidia develop through sporocyst and redia stages in the hepatopancreas of specific snail hosts. The cercariae emerging from the snails then encyst as metacercariae in fish, crabs, or crayfish.

Human disease is usually acquired by ingesting raw, dried, pickled, smoked, or undercooked fish or crabs. The parasites excyst in the duodenum and reach adult size in 1 to 6 weeks. Until recently, treatment of these infections was unsatisfactory, but now praziquantel has proved a very effective remedy. As these infections are widespread in domestic and wild animals, public health control is impractical, and prevention is based on educating people to avoid many of the uncooked or partially cooked traditional dishes of the Orient as well as community-based treatment with praziquantel.

The important liver flukes Asia are *Fasciola hepatica, Clonorchis sinensis,* and *Opisthorchis viverrini.* Clonorchiasis is particularly common in China, and no fewer than 25% of Chinese immigrants in New York are infected.

Fascioliasis

This infection is caused by two large liver flukes, *Fasciola hepatica* and *Fasciola gigantica*.

F. hepatica is common in sheep-raising countries. The adult worm lives in the bile duct of sheep, and eggs are excreted in the feces. Transmission usually occurs when wild watercress contaminated with animal feces is consumed. High prevalence of infection has been reported from Egypt and Bolivia. Some cases are asymptomatic, morbidity being dependent on the intensity and stage of infection.

Clinical Features

Diarrhea, pain in the right hypochondrium, urticaria, fever, coughing, and night sweats together with hepatosplenomegaly, anemia, and a marked eosinophilia occur in the acute phase of infection, about 2 months following ingestion of contaminated watercress or waterplant. Adult flukes in the bile ducts result in cholangitis and cholecystitis, with jaundice and fatty food intolerance.

Diagnosis

Eggs may be found during fecal examination. Various immunodiagnostic assays are available, and they can detect early as well as chronic infections, at a time when few or no eggs are excreted. Ultrasonography, retrograde cholangiopancreatography, and percutaneous cholangiography may be used. Eosinophilia is common.

Treatment

Trichabendazole and nitazoxanide have been found to be effective.

Clonorchiasis
Pathology

Pathological changes are related to the intensity and duration of infection; thousands of adult worms may be found in intrahepatic bile ducts.

Adenomatous hyperplasia and goblet cell metaplasia result in the production of bile with an excessive mucus content. The bile ducts become dilated, tortuous, and thickened; periductal fibrosis may follow. Biliary stasis causes recurrent attacks of E. coli cholangitis. Adenomatous hyperplasia may eventually lead to malignant change, with the development of a mucus secreting cholangiocarcinoma. Liver function usually remains normal. Flukes may also enter the pancreatic ducts and precipitate pancreatitis.

Clinical Features

The period of invasion may be accompanied by a febrile illness with fever, malaise, upper abdominal pain, tender hepatomegaly, and a brisk eosinophilia. Many patients develop no further symptoms until middle age. Heavy infections then produce a vague upper abdominal discomfort, flatulence, and progressive liver enlargement. A curious "hot sensation" over the liver has been described. Other patients present with intermittent bouts of fever, tender hepatomegaly, and jaundice.

Massive infections may lead to obstruction of the common bile duct by flukes; this can result in a state of severe obstructive jaundice. Secondary infection with E. coli often produces a severe illness with rigors, high fever, and pain over the distended liver. Hypoglycemia, salmonellosis, and septic shock may complicate the clinical picture. Victims can also develop biliary calculi, liver abscess, and attacks of acute pancreatitis. Cholangiocarcinomas secondary to clonorchiasis account for 15% of all primary hepatic malignancies in Hong Kong.

Diagnosis

Clonorchiasis is suggested by the triad of classic clinical features, an eosinophilia, and a history of consuming raw or undercooked fish in an endemic region. Identifying eggs in fecal specimens is difficult because of their minute size, and concentration methods are usually required. Clonorchis eggs may also be sought by duodenal aspiration following administration of magnesium sulphate. In order to increase the sensitivity of this important clinical/laboratory test, the duodenal fluid should be filtered through a transparent polycarbonate membrane of 8 micrometer pore size. A transhepatic cholangiogram may reveal curved filling defects or mounds within dilated bile ducts. Ultrasound, endoscopic retrograde cholangiopancreatography (ERCP), computerized tomography (CT), magnetic resonance imaging (MRI), tissue harmonic imaging (THI), immunological, and serological techniques have been used.

Treatment

A total dose of praziquantel 35 to 90 mg per kg bw, divided in 2 doses daily for 2 days, depending on the intensity of infection, resulted in cure rates of 98% to 100% in China.

Opisthorchiasis

Opisthorchis viverrini differs only in minor details from *Clonorchis sinensis*. The main endemic zone is northern Thailand, where the prevalence of infection in the local population may reach 80%. Infection is commonly acquired by eating raw fish in the traditional Thai dish, Koi pla. Community-based education and participation, with partial cost recovery through payment for diagnosis and praziquantel treatment have markedly reduced opisthorchiasis prevalence in northeast Thailand.

Paragonimiasis

Several species of *Paragonimus* infect man. These include *P. westermani* in southeast Asia and India, *P. shriabin* in China, *P. africanus* and *P. uterobilateralis* in west and central Africa, and *P. mexicana* in Central America and South America.

Pathology

Human infection occurs as a result of ingesting raw crabs (or crab sauce) or crayfish, the intermediate hosts for the infective metacercariae stage of the parasite. The immature flukes then penetrate the small intestinal wall and migrate through the peritoneum and diaphragm to the lungs. There, they produce chronic inflammatory and necrotic lesions, forming cysts that may communicate with bronchioles. Aberrant flukes can become encysted in other organs, resulting in eosinophilic abscesses in the intestinal wall, mesentery, liver, spleen, testes, epididymis, subcutaneous tissue, and brain.

Clinical Features

Light infections usually cause no symptoms. The most common manifestation is an early morning cough producing rusty, purulent, or blood-stained sputum that may be flecked with golden brown particles. Occasionally, there may be frank hemoptysis of up to a pint of blood. In contrast with most patients with pulmonary tuberculosis, there is little, if any, deterioration in general health. Physical examination is usually negative. The erythrocyte sedimentation rate (ESR) is usually raised, and there is an eosinophilia. Although a chest x-ray may be normal in 20% of infected patients, the more common abnormalities include a soft "fluffy" shadowing, with or without pleural effusion, linear striations, calcifications, localized pneumothorax, well-defined opacities or nodules with "bubble type" cavities best delineated in tomograms, or a "ring shadow." The apices are seldom affected.

Paragonimiasis can also cause confusing clinical patterns. Abdominal symptoms simulate appendicitis; migratory subcutaneous swellings suggest gnathostomiasis; and a liver abscess can mimic amebiasis. Intracranial cysts can cause epilepsy and/or symptoms of an expanding mass; there may be an associated eosinophilic meningitis, and a skull x-ray may demonstrate calcifications.

Diagnosis

Paragonimiasis is most often misdiagnosed as pulmonary tuberculosis. Helpful differential points are a history of recurrent hemoptysis in an otherwise healthy person who admits to have eaten raw crabs, the x-ray appearances, and an eosinophilia. The diagnosis is confirmed by finding the large, oval, golden brown eggs in the sputum. These may be more obvious in a 24-hour collection to which 3% potassium chloride has been added to dissolve the mucus. They will not be found in sputa stained for tubercle bacilli. Eggs may also be found in the feces or in gastric aspirates.

Treatment

Praziquantel given at 75 mg per kg daily in 3 divided doses for 3 days is an effective therapeutic regimen.

Malnutrition

Individual malnutrition periodically culminates in devastating famines throughout the tropics. More people have starved to death in the past century than at any other time in history, and modern society has been numbed by the television images of skeletal refugees. Life is precarious in the developing world, and if the rains fail or fall too much, if locusts descend or war disrupts distribution systems, hunger is inevitable, and infections flourish.

The most vulnerable victims—usually the young and the very old—present a clinical picture of great variety. At one end of the spectrum are the walking ghosts with marasmus, the victims of rapid, extensive caloric deficiency: in a single word, starvation. At the opposite end are those suffering from chronic protein deficiency, or kwashiorkor. As in most disease states, the majority fall between these classic poles; the clinical picture is further complicated by almost universal infection with multiple parasites and common childhood communicable diseases.

Marasmus

The child with marasmus leaves the impression of an old man's face on an infant's body. There is obvious wasting of muscles with total loss of subcutaneous fat. The buttocks disappear, and the skin is loose and wrinkled.

Scrawny limbs seem incapable of supporting the body. The bony skull appears disproportionately large, and the knees stand out as awkward knobs. Eye lesions are common, and skin rashes with infected "tropical ulcers" are almost universal. Diarrhea is the rule, and complete rectal prolapse from weakness of the anal orifice is not uncommon. A simple measurement of the height and weight on a growth chart will document marked stunting. Nevertheless, the marasmic child is almost surprisingly

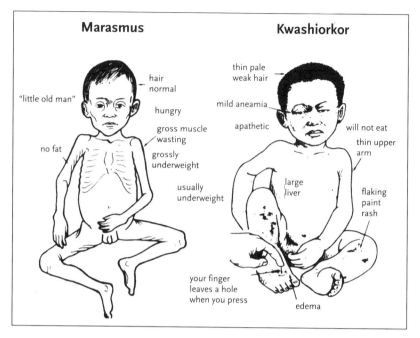

Marasmus   **Kwashiorkor**

hair normal
"little old man"
hungry
no fat
gross muscle wasting
grossly underweight
usually underweight

thin pale weak hair
mild aneamia
apathetic
will not eat
thin upper arm
large liver
flaking paint rash

your finger leaves a hole when you press

edema

FIGURE 33: Clinical faces of malnutrition.

alert, showing constant indications of hunger, such as sucking and grasping movements. They are, however, patently weak and rapidly tire, becoming short of breath after the slightest exertion.

Fat stores are mobilized; glucose uptake by muscle is reduced; and the amino acids, released from tissue breakdown, are used for the resynthesis of other proteins. These adaptions are associated with increased cortisol and diminished insulin activity. Economy is required in the use of resources to maintain processes essential for life. There is a reduction in the basal metabolic rate, cardiac output, and sodium and sweat excretion, and the immune system is compromised.

This clinical picture is usually not due solely to starvation but reflects the added burden of multiple parasitic and respiratory infections. Malaria is extremely common, and measles and tuberculosis are rife in the tropics. Marasmus is very often precipitated, and almost always accompanied by infection, the clinical signs of which may be modified by the profound depression of immunity. Other frequent and often fatal infections include enteritis, monoliasis, generalized herpes simplex, pneumonia, and gram negative septicemia.

Kwashiorkor

In 1933, Cicily Williams, working in west Africa, described a clinical syndrome characterized by edema, dermatosis, a fatty liver, discolored hair, and irritability in children who had to be abruptly weaned from the mother's breast by the arrival of a new baby. She gave the syndrome the name "kwashiorkor," a Ga word that when literally translated means "the sickness of the other child when the next baby is born."

Kwashiorkor is a complex abnormality of metabolism induced by malnutrition. The liver fails to synthesize export proteins such as serum albumin, lipoprotein, and prealbumin, resulting in hypoalbuminemia with generalized edema, gross fatty infiltration of the liver, and a fall in retinol-binding protein that may precipitate vitamin A deficiency. There is cessation of growth, loss of tissue weight, sodium retention, loss of temperature control, and depression of the immune processes, the lymphoid pattern being rather similar to that seen in HIV infection. Kwashiorkor represents a failure of adaption to protein calorie malnutrition and is precipitated when the protein of the diet must be utilized for gluconeogenesis.

Clinical Features

There is nothing subtle about the striking features of kwashiorkor in an African child. Marked edema is usually first seen in the legs, but the face is also affected; the eyes become puffy, and the cheeks droop to give the characteristic "moon face." Edema of the penis may be mistaken for phimosis. The children are apathetic and constantly whining. The hands and feet feel cold, and although obscured by edema, marked muscle wasting can be readily appreciated, especially in the upper arms and around the scapulae. The hair often turns a soft red or white and becomes straight and limp in contrast with the black, crisp, curly hair of the healthy African child.

An "enamel paint" rash is characteristic; it starts as small, purple-stained areas that evolve into black, varnished patches with sharp edges. These coalesce, crack, and peel, leaving desquamated areas resembling burns. The rash is similar in appearance to that of pellagra, but differs in affecting pressure zones, such as the napkin or the inguinal region, knees, elbows, trunk, and trochanteric area. The abdomen is prominent, the liver enlarged, and congestive heart failure (CHF) is often the terminal complication. Xerophthalmia or even keratomalacia may be present. The serum albumin ranges from 0.4 to 2.0 g per 100 ml, and levels >0.8 g per 100 ml carry a poor prognosis.

Treatment

Treatment of these two conditions is similar, and both demand a very high standard of medical and nursing skill to prevent death. Malnutrition is most commonly fatal when it presents in combination with infectious diseases, especially malaria, diarrhea, and respiratory illness. In the tropics, where acute severe malnutrition most commonly occurs, the incidence of these infectious diseases is also high. This has resulted in a highly protocolized management of malnutrition with routine treatment for malaria, intestinal parasites, and bacterial infections being provided.

Ideally, these children should be nursed in a cubicle in which the temperature can be maintained at 80°F to 85°F to guard against hypothermia. A size 20 polyvinyl tube is passed into the stomach via the nose, and 120 to 200 ml per kg bw of half-strength dextrose saline with 2 mg per liter of potassium is administered by continuous drip over 12 to 24 hours. Vitamin deficiencies, including niacin, thiamine, and vitamins C and A, need to be corrected. The blood sugar must be carefully monitored; if it falls to >20 mg per 100 ml, intravenous (IV) glucose and parenteral prednisone are indicated. Active oral feeding should start after 12 to 24 hours, with the goal being 100 kCal containing 4 to 5 g of protein per kg bw daily. The amounts must be gradually increased to the full quota.

It is very important that these feeds be given every 3 hours, day and night. They can be prepared in bulk each morning, divided into eight portions, and stored in a refrigerator. Protein can be provided in dried, skimmed milk or calcium caseinate, sugar as sucrose, and fats as various oils. Small amounts of potassium chloride and magnesium hydroxide are also added. Marasmic children respond slowly, but those with kwashiorkor may respond with a diuresis within a few days, and experience a dramatic return of appetite by the end of the first week.

A fuller diet can then be introduced. The next phase of treatment is equally important; it involves close cooperation with the mother so that a practical diet, which can be maintained during convalescence, can be established. In the absence of a maternal and child service or special "halfway houses," one may be forced to prolong hospital care or witness a rapid relapse.

Maternal and child welfare services, where infants and young children are weighed monthly, is a most effective method of detecting incipient malnutrition. A weight for age chart will visually reveal those who are faltering, and dietary supplements can be offered. There is some evidence that overly aggressive refeeding, especially with inappropriate foods, can complicate recovery. For example, malaria outbreaks have occurred in refugee camps after foods high in para amino benzoic acid and vitamin E are introduced.

The management of malnutrition presents clinicians with a complex clinical problem that is fundamentally social in origin. Poverty, high food prices, government manipulation of food supplies, poor maternal education, and co-existing pathologies all contribute to the incidence of malnutrition. Practitioners in developing countries will commonly encounter malnourished children, and isolated cases can be managed in existing facilities. However, epidemic malnutrition in the context of famine requires vast budgets and logistic capacities, and is often the largest component of humanitarian aid operations. In either case, the role of the physician should be extended beyond individual clinical management; one must, for example, investigate why a particular child is malnourished and whether this may apply to other community members. Poverty and lack of education may prompt a different response to soaring food prices or lack of access to food because of conflict.

Current guidelines for treatment of malnutrition use a framework of Community Management of Acute Malnutrition (CMAM), which emphasizes the role of ready-to-use foods in home feeding to allow rapid discharge of patients from feeding centers. This shift away from long admissions to in-patient therapeutic feeding centers recognizes the problems caused by admitting a child along with a mother as caregiver for several weeks, which frequently leads to neglect of other previously well children left at home. Feeding centers should be monitored for cure rates, failure rates, mortality rates, and length of stay, and should be striving to achieve targets for all these indicators. Active case finding and community screening will help to build a more complete picture of the effectiveness of a malnutrition program.

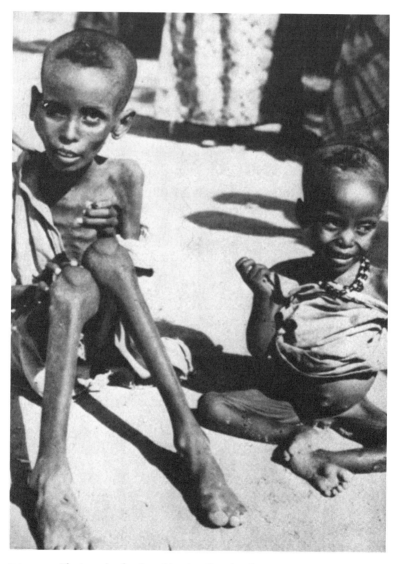

FIGURE 34: The tragedy of malnutrition in a Somali refugee camp is seen in classic marasmus (left) and kwashiorkor (right).

Hereditary Anemias

Anemia remains one of the most important medical problems of the tropics and subtropics. When relatively mild, it reduces the physical well being and work capacity of whole populations; when severe, it is an important cause of death. Common diseases already considered include malnutrition, with deficient intake of iron often compounded by hookworm infection; infections, especially malaria; hypersplenism; and nutritional deficiency of folate and vitamin B12, which may be compounded by intestinal malabsorption. Other major causes of anemia include the genetic disorders, which are prevalent wherever *P. falciparum* malaria is endemic. The hereditary anemias of the tropics and subtropics constitute the most numerous and important examples of human hereditary genetic defects. Hundreds of millions of people are born each year with these abnormal traits.

Physiology

Molecules of hemoglobin consist of four peptide chains, each chain being associated with a heme group. In extrauterine life, these are alpha, beta, gamma, and delta chains, and each hemoglobin molecule contains a pair of alpha chains and a pair of another type. The physiological hemoglobins so formed are:

1. HbF, or fetal hemoglobin, consists of two alpha chains and two gamma chains. This is the major hemoglobin synthesized from the eighth week of gestation; while synthesis normally ceases at birth, HbF is still found in decreasing amounts until the third month of extrauterine life.
2. HbA, or adult hemoglobin, which in extrauterine life, largely replaces HbF. It is composed of two alpha chains and two beta chains.

3. HbA$_2$ is composed of two alpha chains and two delta chains. It normally does not exceed 3.5% of normal hemoglobin.

The synthesis of each of these chains is controlled by one or more genes. Thus, on chromosome 16, there are two alpha genes per haploid genome, while the other globin chains are controlled by single genes clustered on chromosome 11. There are two main groups of inherited disorders of hemoglobin production.

1. Deficient production of one of the globin chains: the thalassemias
2. Structural hemoglobin variants in which there is substitution of one amino acid for another in one of the globin chains: the hemoglobinopathies

The Thalassemias

The thalassemias are a heterogeneous group of disorders resulting from a reduced synthesis rate of one or more of the globin chains of the hemoglobin molecule. Most of the clinical features of the more common thalassemias are due to the unbalanced globin chain synthesis, the excess partner chains being precipitated in red cell precursors. These disorders occur worldwide, but the highest prevalence is in a broad band stretching from the Mediterranean to southern China.

Beta Thalassemia

Two allelomorphic genes on chromosome 11 normally code the beta globin chains. Beta thalassemia results from a variety of point mutations in these genes, leading to deficiencies in messenger RNA coding for the beta globin chain of adult hemoglobin. Some of these mutations result in no synthesis of the chains (B°) while others lead to reduced synthesis (B$^+$).

Beta Thalassemia Major represents the homozygous state when both genes on chromosome 11 are affected (B°B°). Nonproduction of the beta globin chains results in precipitation of highly unstable alpha chains. This prevents normal maturation and release of red cell precursors from the bone marrow. The synthesis of gamma chains persists beyond the neonatal period, with these chains binding to excess alpha chains. The pathological results of this are as follows:

1. A severe anemia with HbF accounting for 80% to 90% of the hemoglobin. HbF, which is heterogeneously distributed among the red cells, has a high oxygen affinity; this, together with the marked anemia, produces a severe degree of anoxia of the tissues.

2. The anoxia stimulates erythropoietin production and expansion of the bone marrow in an almost neoplastic fashion. The end result is erosion of bone with distortion and thinning of the cortex, the development of paravertebral tumors, and wasting.

3. Gross enlargement of the spleen associated with increased plasma volume and cardiomegaly.

4. Increased intestinal absorption of iron causing liver damage, multiple endocrine disorders, and cardiomyopathy. Patients require blood transfusion every 6 weeks, and this further accentuates the iron overload.

Beta Thalassemia Intermedia is the homologous state causing disease of insufficient severity to require regular blood transfusion. The hemoglobin concentration remains between 7 to 10.5 g per 100 ml. This clinical syndrome may arise from inheritance of B^+ genes, through coinheritance of alpha thalassemia, or due to hereditary persistence of HbF (HPFH).

Beta Thalassemia Minor is the heterozygous state with only one of the beta genes being affected. Heterozygotes for the B^+ gene are not anemic, and those for the B^o gene, only mildly so, although their hemoglobin concentrations may fall during pregnancy or with an infection. Blood films may be hypochromic and microcytic, but unless there is a coexistent iron deficiency, iron stores will be normal. The hallmarks of this condition are inappropriately low levels of MCV and MCH when compared with the hemoglobin concentration. Hemoglobin electrophoresis will reveal a concentration of HbA_2 greater than 4%.

Clinical Features

The child with thallesemia remains well during the first 3 to 4 months of life and then fails to thrive, developing fever, anorexia, recurrent respiratory, and gastrointestinal infections. The abdomen becomes distended by a rapidly enlarging spleen, and bone marrow hyperplasia is reflected in skull bossing and a "mongoloid facies." The red cells are hypochromic, and there are numerous target cells. The hemoglobin is 3 to 5 g per 100 ml, and electrophoresis shows that 80% to 90% is HbF. These children rapidly die unless treated by regular blood transfusion.

However, while transfusion transiently restores a viable clinical state, complications of iron overload are likely to appear in adolescence. These include stunted growth, lack of muscle tissue, failure of sexual maturity, evidence of hypoparathyroid or adrenal cortical dysfunction, and diabetes. Until recently, most victims died between 16 and 24 years of age due to a cardiac arrhythmia or recurrent heart failure.

Treatment

In early childhood, the standard approach has been based on a hypertransfusion regimen maintaining a hemoglobin concentration of 10 to 14 g per 100 ml by blood administration every 6 weeks. A supertransfusion regimen in which the hemoglobin is maintained at 14 to 15 g per 100 ml has given better results, with more effective suppression of endogenous erythropoiesis, shrinkage of bone marrow, and a greater reduction in iron absorption without increasing the long-term requirement for transfused red blood cells. If available, only young red cells with a prolonged survival time should be used. Either regimen must include chelation therapy. Desferrioxamine flenters cells only briefly and is cleared from the body within 6 hours; to obtain optimal chelation, this drug is administered by continuous 8 to 12 hour subcutaneous infusion in a dose of 1,500 to 2,000 mg, up to 5 nights weekly. Vitamin C is also a chelating agent, but it can cause increased iron deposition in cardiac muscle. Splenectomy may be required in children developing hypersplenism.

There have been several new therapeutic developments that are still being assessed. Bone marrow transplantation from an HLA identical sibling may give a complete cure; prognosis is determined by the amount of chelation of iron up to the point of transplantation. Azacytidine increases gamma globin synthesis, but its use has been limited because it is carcinogenic in animals. Finally, modifications of standard surgical approaches offer new hope; partial splenic embolism appears to offer the same benefits as total splenectomy without incurring the equivalent risk of infection and the need for life-long antibiotic prophylaxis.

Alpha Thalassemia

Four genes on chromosome 16 (aa/aa) code for the alpha globin chains. Alpha thalassemia results from deletion of one or more of these genes or, much less commonly, through point mutations. Because the alpha chains of HbA and HbF are under the same genetic control, there is defective production of both these hemoglobins. The gamma and the beta chains are produced at a normal rate, but due to the lack of alpha chains, they form tetramers: Hb Barts (Y4) in uterine life, and HbH (B4) after birth. These tetramers are stable enough to allow the red cell precursors to mature and be delivered into the circulation. The degree of ineffective erythropoiesis is, therefore, less than in beta thalassemia, but the life span of mature red cells is reduced. In addition, because of their high oxygen affinity, these tetramers are useless as oxygen carriers.

Clinical Features

Deletion of one gene (− a/aa) is common in most tropical populations and causes no overt clinical abnormality. Deletion of 2 genes (− a/ − a or − − /aa) leads to a mild anemia with inappropriately reduced values for MCV and MCH. Deletion of the two genes on the same chromosome is largely confined to Asian and Mediterranean populations. These "defects," in fact, carry certain advantages because they give some protection against severe malaria, and when coinherited with beta thalassemia, reduce the severity of the latter condition. No treatment is usually required, but it is important that the blood picture not be misinterpreted as being due to iron deficiency anemia.

Deletion of 3 genes coding for the alpha globin chains (− − / − a) causes hemoglobin H disease, a moderately severe hemolytic anemia. In Thailand and surrounding regions, coinheritance of an abnormal hemoglobin in which the alpha chain is affected—hemoglobin Constant

Spring—has the same effect as deletion of alpha genes. In affected neo-nates, as many as 25% of the hemoglobin is HbH. Adult patients experi-ence a varying degree of anemia, the hemoglobin in the steady state being about 8 to 10 g per 100 ml, falling as low as 4 g per 100 ml during pregnancy. The spleen is enlarged. A blood film will reveal hypo-chromia and microcytosis as well as variations in size and shape of red cells and target cells. Staining for reticulocytes with brilliant cresyl blue will reveal inclusion bodies in erythrocytes; on electrophoresis, an abnormal, fast-moving hemoglobin accounts for as much as 25% of the total. In patients with the alpha thalassemia Constant Spring abnormal-ity, electrophoresis will reveal an additional band between that of HbA$_2$ and the origin. These patients may require transfusion when the hemo-globin falls as in pregnancy.

When there is deletion of all 4 genes ($-\ -/-\ -$), the only hemo-globin that can be synthesized in the second half of fetal life is Hb Barts (Y4), which is not an effective carrier of oxygen to the tissues. This condition, known as the "Hemoglobin Barts hydrops syndrome," results in a severely anemic, edematous fetus, which either dies late in preg-nancy or immediately after birth. The mother is also brought into jeopardy due to a high incidence of toxemia, obstructed labor, or post-partum hemorrhage.

Hemoglobinopathies

The hemoglobinopathies are inherited conditions in which abnormal hemoglobins with one or more structural changes, usually a single amino acid substitution in a globin chain, are synthesized at a normal or near normal rate. As with the thalassemias, inheritance is through paired allelomorphic genes, and may be homozygous or heterozygous. The most important of these abnormal hemoglobins is sickle cell hemo-globin (HbS).

Sickle cell hemoglobin (HbS) differs from normal adult hemoglobin (HbA) by a valine residue replacing glutamic acid in the sixth position on the beta globin chain. The amino acid substitution does not effect the oxygenated form of HbS but, when the concentration of deoxyge-nated HbS is sufficiently great, molecules polymerize into filaments. These associate laterally to form bundles of fibers, which distort the red cell into a sickle shape, leading to their premature destruction and anemia. More importantly, these abnormally shaped cells increase the viscosity of deoxygenated blood, impeding flow through capillaries. As oxygen levels fall, the body responds by increased sickling of cells, which can completely block the vessels. The effects of the anemia are ameliorated in that HbS has a low oxygen affinity, which enhances oxygen release. It is, therefore, not the chronic anemia but rather the mechanical impedance to blood flow caused by the sickled cells that is the most important factor in this disease.

Sickle Cell Anemia is the homozygous state in which 90% of the hemoglobin is HbS. The more important pathological abnormalities are:

Anemia: There is a chronic hemolytic anemia with a hemoglobin concentration in the steady state of 7 to 9 g per 100 ml, a reticulocytosis of 10% to 12%, and a serum bilirubin of 2 mg per 100 ml. Episodes of severe anemia occur due to sequestration of red cells in the spleen, increases in the rate of hemolysis, and temporary aplasia following parvovirus infections.

Vasoocclusive incidents: Blood vessel blockage may occur anywhere in the body. Bones are commonly involved, and infarction may be complicated by Salmonella osteomyelitis. The most severe occlusive incidents are those affecting the brain, lungs, liver, mesentery, and spleen.

Spleen: The spleen at first enlarges, but by the age of 10, it usually is atrophic. Splenic function is compromised long before the organ recedes, and these children are at risk for severe pneumococcal infection. In other individuals, the spleen may remain large and produce the signs and symptoms of hypersplenism.

Clinical Features

The course of sickle cell anemia is that of a chronic mild to moderate hemolytic anemia, punctuated by various blood or vasoocclusive "crises." These may occur at any age. Usually the child appears normal during the first 3 to 4 months of life and then fails to thrive. They are pale, sometimes jaundiced, with hepatosplenomegaly and bossing of the skull. A common vasoocclusive episode at this stage is the "hand-foot syndrome," in which there is pain and swelling of either hand or foot associated with fever and a leukocytosis. Two common causes of death in the first 3 years of life are an overwhelming pneumococcal infection and the splenic sequestration syndrome. Both complications erupt suddenly: the former often presenting as coma, and the latter as a life-threatening anemia associated with acute enlargement of the spleen.

Sickle cell children between the ages of 3 and 10 tend to remain unwell. They are anemic, weak, thin, and at risk for repeated infections. They present a characteristic picture with widely separated eyes, depressed bridge of the nose, irregular growth of the fingers, long arms, upper dorsal kyphosis, and bossing of the skull. They suffer episodes of severe hemolytic anemia with a high reticulocytosis and jaundice. They develop marrow aplasia following parvovirus infection, and reticulo- cytes disappear from the peripheral blood. Vasoocclusive episodes may be recurrent, often involving the long bones with severe pain, local swelling, and fever; areas of necrosis may be complicated by *Salmonella* osteomyelitis. Infarctive episodes may occur anywhere in the body as "painful crises." Other attacks mimic acute appendicitis, or when the brain is affected, produce convulsions, sudden paralysis, or coma. There is an inability to concentrate urine, and these children may suffer from enuresis as well as episodes of hematuria. A mild to moderate cardio- megaly is often accompanied by flow murmurs. Toward the end of this period, recurrent chronic disabling leg ulcerations may develop.

Adolescence is often delayed. Following puberty, males become prone to recurrent attacks of painful nocturnal priapism lasting 2 to 6 hours. Other painful crises continue to occur. An acute chest syndrome may present with pleuritic pain, with or without a cough; at first, no abnormal clinical or radiological signs may be found, but a syndrome evolves with fever, breathlessness, cyanosis, and respiratory failure associated with bilateral basilar dullness and rales. Another typical pat- tern is the "girdle syndrome," which starts with pain in the lumbar region followed by rapid clinical deterioration, a silent distended abdo- men, and respiratory failure.

Individuals surviving into adult life may remain almost symptom- free or may continue to be subject to painful crises; occasionally, pul- monary and girdle crises. By this time, most develop gall stones that may give rise to duct obstruction. The spleen has usually atrophied, but sequestration crises may be associated with acute hepatomegaly. Pregnancy once posed a great danger because unless precautions were taken, there was a 50% fetal wastage and a maternal mortality approaching 30%. These rates have now been significantly reduced in most parts of the world.

Finally, as survivors pass into their fourth or fifth decades, they are liable to develop severe pyelonephritis or chronic hyperuricemia with gouty arthritis. A retinopathy, in which multiple comma-shaped capillary segments are seen with closed afferent and efferent vessels, is associated with intraocular hemorrhage, retinal detachment, and blindness.

Despite these common clinical patterns, sickle cell anemia is not a homogeneous condition. Several different mutations are now recognized, and associated inheritance of alpha thalassemia and the gene coding for HPFH have a considerable ameliorating effect. Thus, individuals with sickle cell anemia in eastern Saudi Arabia and India are less seriously affected. Environmental factors are also probably important; adults with sickle cell anemia in the Caribbean appear to do remarkably well, while those in the colder climatic conditions seem more prone to severe or fatal crises.

Diagnosis

Blood films often reveal irreversibly sickled red cells as well as crenated or fragmented erythrocytes. Howell Jolly bodies are an indication of splenic atrophy. There is a varying reticulocytosis, mean 15%, and most patients have a neutrophil leukocytosis, which during a crisis may rise to high levels. The mean serum bilirubin is 2.0 mg per 100 ml. The sickling test carried out with freshly prepared sodium metabisulphite reveals rapid generalized sickling, and electrophoresis of hemoglobin on cellulose acetate membranes confirms that 90% of the hemoglobin is HbS. Sickle cell anemia in India and Saudi Arabia is associated with a raised concentration of HbF.

Treatment

Few affected children survive to adolescence childhood in rural Africa. In other regions, including Africa, where medical facilities are more freely available, much can be done to ensure that HbS patients live to lead active adult lives. It is important that the diagnosis be made at birth by screening umbilical cord blood so that parents can be counseled and advised on management. Chemoprophylaxis against malaria and pneumococcal infection should start at 3 months, and intramuscular (IM) long-acting penicillin is often preferable to daily oral administration. Prophylactic immunization schedules should be rigorously followed.

Acute splenic sequestration requires emergency blood transfusion, and if recurrent, splenectomy. An aplastic crisis can be treated by outpatient transfusion. The dangers of transfusions in many parts of the world must be appreciated. Forty-three percent of children with sickle cell anemia in the Ivory Coast who had been given more than two transfusions were HIV1- or HIV2-positive. Transfusions should be given only as a life saving measure unless the blood can be adequately screened.

Minor crises can be treated by bed rest, warmth, hydration, and analgesics, while life threatening crises may require emergency total exchange transfusions. Exchange blood transfusion is also indicated for patients with central nervous system (CNS) involvement and renal failure, during pregnancy, and before any major operation. Splenectomy may be indicated in a minority of patients with persisting splenomegaly and hypersplenism.

Other Causes of Sickle Cell Disease

Clinical and pathological features, similar but usually milder than those seen in sickle cell anemia (SS), occur in individuals who have co-inherited the sickle cell gene with either the gene for hemoglobin C (SC), or that of B° thalassemia (SB°). SC disease, endemic in west Africa, is often very mild. However, some individuals may be severely affected, suffering from periodic painful crises, and during pregnancy, from a major crisis. Avascular necrosis of the head of the femur is said to be five times as common in SC disease as in SS. Another hazard for these individuals is that flight in under-pressurized aircraft may precipitate splenic infarction. The diagnosis is confirmed by demonstrating two major abnormal bands on hemoglobin electrophoresis. Sickle cell-B° thalassemia closely resembles SS disease, but is usually milder, the concentration of HbS being only 60% to 65%. The differential diagnosis is confirmed by finding a HbA_2 concentration $<4\%$, low MCV and MCH indices, and an elevated concentration of HbF.

Sickle Cell Trait is the heterozygous state (AS) in which 25% to 45% of the hemoglobin is HbS, and the remainder HbA. There may be some defect in urinary concentration and occasional hematuria. Exposure to intense cold can precipitate a major crisis, but the vast majority of these individuals suffer no ill effects, and they enjoy partial protection from severe *P. falciparum* malaria.

Glucose 6 Phosphate Dehydrogenase Deficiency (G6PD Deficiency)

There are some 400 allelic variants of glucose 6 phosphate dehydrogenases, enzymes that catalyze the initial step in the anaerobic hexose monophosphate oxidation of glucose. The red cells require the redox potential generated by this reaction to combat oxidative stress. Some of these enzymes are defective, and individuals inheriting them may react to oxidative stress by episodes of acute hemolysis. Inheritance of the enzymes is coded for by a single recessive gene on the X chromosome. Thus, the expression of a defective enzyme might be expected only in hemizygous males and homozygous females. However, female heterozygotes may also be affected because of random inactivation of one X chromosome.

The following polymorphic variants are important in the tropics and subtropics. The severely deficient ($<10\%$ activity) is found in the Mediterranean, north Africa, western Asia, and the Indian subcontinent, as well as in southeast Asia, China, Korea, and Oceania (G6PD Mediterranean and G6PD Union). Two moderately severely deficient variants (10% to 60% activity) are found in southeast Asia, China, Korea, and Oceania (G6PD Mahidol and G6PD Canton), and a third moderately severely deficient variant is found in sub-Saharan Africa (G6PD A-). Gd Mali achieves local polymorphic frequency in sub-Saharan Africa ($<10\%$ activity), resulting in intermittent hemolysis.

Clinical Features

G6PD deficiency is the most common cause of severe neonatal jaundice in some regions where deficiency is common. These children, whose immature livers cannot deal with the hyperbilirubinemia, become severely jaundiced although this may not be readily appreciated in dark-skinned infants. Delay in recognition may be followed by kernicterus. Other patients suffer attacks of acute hemolysis and jaundice, mainly as a result of exposure to oxidant drugs or certain infections. A few days later, a reticulocytosis sets in, and spontaneous recovery occurs over a period of about 1 month. Severe episodes are liable to be complicated by acute renal failure.

The African enzyme G6PD A- is active in young red cells but becomes immature as the red cell ages. In the steady state, its activity is about 15% of normal. Attacks are of varying severity and are precipitated by oxidant drugs, such as primaquine; and by infections, particularly typhoid, pneumonia, and viral hepatitis. Attacks associated with the Canton enzyme are precipitated in a similar manner to the African variety but tend to be more severe. The activity of the G6PD Mediterranean enzyme is <10%, and episodes of very severe hemolysis are often followed by acute renal failure, especially in adults. One precipitating stress is hypersensitivity to fava beans (*Vicia fava*) or to the verbena plant. Attacks do not occur with every contact; indeed, an individual may suffer only a single attack during a lifetime, and on occasion, attacks occur when there is no history of exposure.

Epidemiological, clinical, parasitological, and in vitro evidence is available that demonstrates the protective effect of G6PD deficiency against severe *P. falciparum* malaria.

Diagnosis

This condition should be suspected in any patient from Africa, the Mediterranean, the Middle East, southeast Asia, or the Caribbean who presents with an acute hemolytic anemia. The urine contains hemoglobin, and the red cells have a characteristic "bitten out" appearance. The Coomb's test is negative. A fluorescent spot test on dried blood on filter paper is both sensitive and specific. Further confirmation may be given by various dye tests for quantitative methemoglobin reduction. In the

Caribbean and southeast Asia, screening of the umbilical cord blood of neonates is practiced routinely. The various enzymes may be identified by electrophoresis and enzyme kinetic studies.

Treatment

Provided the diagnosis is made sufficiently early, neonates usually respond well to phototherapy, but some may require exchange transfusion. Many attacks in older patients are mild and require no treatment. Blood transfusion should be used only when anemia is life threatening or associated with acute renal failure. The latter complication often responds to medical measures, but some patients require dialysis.

Familial Mediterranean Fever

This puzzling hereditary disorder, transmitted through autosomal recessive genes, affects Sephardic Jews and other groups living in the Mediterranean basin. Multiple family members may experience recurrent brief attacks of acute endothelial inflammation. The most frequent presentation is a sudden sharp periumbilical pain spreading across the abdomen, and associated with fever and leukocytosis. The pain and temperature reach a peak after 6 hours and gradually subside to normal within 1 day. Less-common manifestations are synovitis, arthritis, and pleurisy; late complications include amyloidosis and bowel strangulation secondary to chronic adhesions. The prompt use of colchicine can arrest an attack, and a dose of 1.0 to 1.5 mg daily can prevent recurrent episodes.

Miscellaneous

Tropical Tumors

Several important malignant tumors occur in tropical settings. These include the following.

Burkitt's Lymphoma

In the late 1950s, Dennis Burkitt, an Irish surgeon working in Uganda with O'Connor and Davies, described an endemic form of B cell lymphoma affecting the jaws of children. It is now recognized as the most common childhood cancer in subequatorial Africa and in Papua New Guinea; rare cases have been reported from countries around the world.

Pathology

Burkitt's lymphoma is found primarily in the bones of the jaw and in the ovaries of young girls. Undifferentiated lymphoblasts surround scattered large clear histiocytes, giving a "starry sky" appearance under low-power microscopy. The tumors are commonly multiple, symmetrical, and extremely fast growing, with a cell doubling time of only 24 hours. They reach an enormous size within a matter of days. These tumors also occur in the kidneys, retroperitoneal tissues, thyroid, distal long bones, breast, testes, and parotid glands. The pathogenesis of Burkitt's lymphoma is not altogether clear, but it involves a complex relationship among

Chronic *P. falciparum* infection

Persistent Epstein-Barr virus (EBV) infection

Chromosomal translocations in B lymphocytes with deregulation of the oncogenic c − myc gene

Clinical Features

The most common presentation is a young child with a unilateral or bilateral facial swelling. Some children are first seen by a dentist because of loosening of deciduous molar teeth. A maxillary tumor may obliterate the antrum, and the palate bulges downward. The tumor may also spread upward into the orbit, causing proptosis and destruction of the eye. Pain is seldom severe, and the cervical lymph nodes are not involved. X-ray of the jaw reveals osteolytic lesions with erosion round the roots of the teeth. In northern Nigeria, large ovarian tumors develop in girls ages 10 to 16. A less-common presenting symptom is a flaccid paraplegia due to extension of a retroperitoneal tumor.

Diagnosis and Treatment

The diagnosis is confirmed either by biopsy or aspiration of tumor material. In view of the rapid growth of these tumors, treatment is urgent, and 80% to 90% of these patients will respond initially to aggressive cytotoxic therapy. Large abdominal tumors should be removed surgically. Despite periods of remission, relapses occur in 60% of cases. Relapses within 3 months seldom respond to further chemotherapy, but those occurring after this period respond well. A 70% cure rate may be expected in African children with only jaw involvement. Important complications of cytotoxic drug treatment are hyperkalemia and hyperuricemia with acute renal failure.

Nasopharyngeal Carcinoma

Nasopharyngeal carcinoma is more than 10 to 20 times as common in southern Chinese as in Europeans. As with Burkitt's lymphoma, this tumor appears to be associated with EBV infection. EBV can be detected in tumor cells, and serological titers for EBV antibodies are directly proportional to the amount of tumor present. The clinical presentation is varied and often confusing. Common manifestations include obstruction of the Eustachian or nasal passages, cervical lymphadenopathy, persistent neuralgic facial pain, cranial nerve palsies, and proptosis due to orbital involvement. The small primary lesion in the post-nasal space is frequently not recognized until later complications emerge. Radiotherapy is often successful, but patients with cranial nerve palsies or cervical lymph node involvement have a poor prognosis.

Kaposi's Sarcoma

Yet another tumor, which may or may not be secondary to a viral infection, is the endemic Kaposi's sarcoma of central Africa and Papua New Guinea, where it accounts for 9% of recorded malignancies. The "epicenter" of endemicity in Africa is in eastern Zaire. Kaposi's sarcoma is also a major complication of HIV/AIDS.

Pathology

In African men, Kaposi's sarcoma is a very slowly progressive disease of the extremities, characterized by purple nodules and local edema. Early in the course of the disease, the histologic picture consists of dilated, thin-walled vascular spaces with jagged outlines, sparsely infiltrated with lymphocytes and plasma cells. Later, there is spindle cell proliferation with frequent mitosis. The steady growth of these lesions, the limited geographical distribution, and the association with immunodeficiency have suggested a viral origin.

Clinical Features

There are two peaks of incidence: the first in children of either sex, ages 2 to 3 years; and the second in adult men. In children, the usual presentation is with a highly malignant lymphoma characterized by general enlargement of lymph nodes, visceral involvement, and early death but with no skin lesions. In adults, the mean age of presentation is 40 years. The lesions tend to be multiple and symmetrical, affecting primarily the legs, and less commonly, arms or genitalia. The first symptom is usually edema of one or both legs, followed by macular patches, and then slowly growing purplish or hyperpigmented nodules or plaques.

Spontaneous remission may occur but in other individuals, after a period of years, the nodules grow rapidly, become confluent, and ulcerate to form florid tumors. Other patients develop a woody infiltration of the whole limb with enlargement of regional lymph nodes. Early visceral involvement often remains asymptomatic, with raspberry-like lesions seen on the palate or in the gastrointestinal tract, or as pulmonary nodules on chest x-ray. Terminally, however, there may be gross loss of weight, pulmonary consolidation, and bilateral pleural effusion.

Diagnosis and Treatment

The diagnosis depends on the characteristic clinical and histological features. Early lesions respond well to radiotherapy, and later lesions to cytotoxic drug therapy, although aggressive chemotherapy in HIV/AIDS-infected patients may precipitate fatal opportunistic infection by further depleting the patient's immunological capacity.

Snake Bite

Tens of thousands of people die or are permanently crippled from snake bite each year in the tropics despite the fact that early treatment with modern antivenoms is highly effective. Surprisingly, when venomous snakes bite humans, venom is injected on only about 50% of occasions possibly because the venom apparatus is at a mechanical disadvantage when the snake strikes at a human hand or foot when inadvertently trodden upon or picked up. The doctor should, therefore, observe the patient for the development of systemic signs before treating with an expensive and a potentially dangerous antivenom.

The venom secreting glands of snakes are connected by ducts to grooved or canalized fangs situated in the upper jaw. When biting or striking, the glands are compressed by surrounding muscles so that the venom is squeezed out through the fang. Venoms are clear fluids of complex chemical structure, containing toxic and nontoxic enzymes, proteins, and peptides evolved rapidly to immobilize and help digest the prey. Of the approximately 2,500 known species of snakes, more than 300 are capable of killing humans. These are classified as follows.

Viperidae

Vipers, Adders, and Moccasins
These snakes are relatively short, measuring 20 cm to (exceptionally) nearly 4 meters in length. They have a relatively stout, flattened body,

distinctive neck, and a triangle-shaped head covered with numerous small rough scales. They possess long, tubular, mobile fangs that are folded back against the maxilla in the resting position, but that come forward into an erect position when the snake strikes. Species of medical importance include the saw-scaled or carpet vipers of Africa and Asia, the puff adders of Africa, and Russell's vipers of India, Burma, and southeast Asia.

One group of vipers, the pit vipers, has a thermosensitive pit between the eye and the nostril; Malayan pit vipers and the rattlesnakes and moccasins of America are examples. Snakes are usually well camouflaged and are easily trodden on by people walking barefoot along forest paths or working in the fields, rubber plantations, or rice paddies.

Clinical Features. Viper venoms cause both local and systemic reactions. If venom is injected, the bite is painful and is soon followed by local swelling, the extent of which is probably related to the dose of venom injected. Swelling normally becomes maximum within 1 to 2 days of the bite. The area may then become brawny and indurated with ecchymosis and blisters often containing blood. Some venoms can cause local tissue necrosis through direct cytotoxic, digestive enzyme activity, and secondary to damage of the vascular endothelium, resulting in ischemia. Gangrene rarely results from arterial thrombosis.

Dead tissue may become secondarily infected. Systemically, procoagulant effects of many of these venoms cause disseminated intravascular coaqulopathy (DIC), resulting in fibrinogen consumption and consequently incoagulable blood. Hemorrhagic venom components cause damage to the basement membrane of the capillary endothelium, causing endothelial disorganization that results in systemic bleeding at different sites throughout the body. Systemic envenoming may therefore present with bleeding gums, epistaxis, diffuse ecchymoses, hematuria, melena, and/or incoagulable blood.

Soon after the bite, the patient may suffer severe hypotension caused by potent vasodilators present in the venom. By the time the seriously envenomed patient reaches hospital, they may be nauseated, vomiting, and even in profound hypovolemic shock. In some cases, the blood does not clot although the platelet count may be normal. There is a

neutrophil leukocytosis and severe anemia due to the action of hemorrhagic components present in the venom. Shock may occur at this
stage, which may lead to acute renal failure. A complication, particularly associated with Russell's viper bites, is pituitary hemorrhage,
which may present initially as acute hypoglycemia with later features
of hypothyroidism and hypogonadism.

Management. First aid treatment should be limited to immobilizing
the whole patient and especially the bitten limb. Tourniquets should
never be recommended because they will cause ischemia and gangrene
and will aggravate local effects of the venom. Pressure immobilization
with a crepe bandage is also contraindicated in bites by most vipers
whose venom causes local swelling and necrosis. This compression
exacerbates local effects of envenoming and raises the pressure in tight
fascial compartments in the limbs with the risk of serious ischemia.
The patient should be kept calm and should be taken to hospital as
rapidly as possible even if no signs of envenoming are initially apparent.
If there is little local swelling, it is unlikely that serious envenoming
has occurred, and an agitated patient may be reassured. Systemic
envenoming following bites by vipers is suggested by bleeding from the
gums caused by the action of venom hemorrhagins, or of old wounds
caused by fibrinolysis. A simple test—a 20-minute whole blood–
clotting test—is performed by placing 1 to 2 ml of venous blood in a
new, clean, dry test tube or other glass vessel, leaving it undisturbed
for 20 minutes and then observing whether it has clotted by tipping
the vessel; nonclotting after this time indicates venom-induced consumption coagulopathy.

Antivenom should be given only to patients with signs of systemic
envenoming (shock, bleeding, incoagulable blood) or to those with
severe local envenoming (rapidly evolving or massive swelling, especially involving digits). It is important to know the identity of the snake
responsible for the bite so that an appropriate and specific antivenom
can be used and complications, such as acute renal failure following
Russell's viper bites, may be anticipated. However, identification of the
snake is frequently difficult due to the unreliability of the patient's
description; likewise, doctors are often untrained in snake identification. Diagnostic ELISA kits for the detection of specific venoms are

available only in Australia (CSL Venom Detection Kit). Such kits are simply not available in developing countries. If the snake cannot be identified, a polyvalent/specific antivenom covering the venoms of the important species in that geographical area should be used. Great care should be taken in handling even a dead snake because powerful reflexes can result in the injection of venom even after the death of the animal.

Antivenom is administered either diluted 2 to 3 times in normal saline and delivered by slow intravenous (IV) infusion drip over 30 to 60 minutes, by slow IV "push," or by a bolus injection at 2 ml per minute. The drip is started at 10 drops per minute and gradually increased to 150 drops per minute, provided that an anaphylactoid reaction does not develop. To counteract this, adrenaline must be available in the syringe before the start of antivenom administration; in the event of a reaction, the antivenom should be stopped, and 0.5 ml of 1:1000 adrenaline given intramuscularly (IM). After the reaction has subsided, the remainder of the antivenom should be given under antihistamine cover. The dose of antivenom for children is the same as for adults. The effect of the antivenom may be evident within 1 to 2 hours, but the dose may have to be repeated if, for example, the blood remains incoagulable 6 hours after the start of antivenom. If a local necrotic lesion develops, the patient should be treated with appropriate antibiotics, and the immunity of the patient should be boosted with antitetanus toxoid unless he was previously unimmunized. Surgical debridement and subsequent skin grafting may occasionally be necessary.

Elapidae

Cobras, Mambas, Kraits, Coral Snakes, Australian/New Guinean Taipans, Black and Brown Snakes, and Death Adders
Cobras are relatively long snakes, often more than 2 meters long; king cobras may grow to more than 6 meters in length. They are easily recognized by their habit of rearing up and extending the hood behind the neck when defending themselves. They possess short, nonmobile, grooved fangs situated at the front of the upper jaw. The Elapidae group includes the cobras of India, Africa, and southeast Asia, the kraits of southeast Asia, the coral snakes of the New World, the mambas of

Africa, and all the Australasian venomous snakes. Although vipers are mainly concentrated in the fields and forests, snakes such as cobras are attracted to human habitations in search of prey, such as rats. They often enter houses at night where they coil up in receptacles, cupboards, or dark corners, remaining unseen until disturbed. Kraits also enter human dwellings at night in search of their prey. Bites often occur when the people sleeping on the ground move in their sleep, thus alarming the snake.

Clinical Features. Immediately after a bite by a cobra, there may be a burning sensation at the site of the bite. The venom of most cobras causes local necrosis. The main life-threatening danger is systemic neurotoxic envenoming. Cobra venoms bind postsynaptically to the acetylcholine receptor sites on the motor end plates, producing an effect similar to that of curare. The first sign of poisoning is often ptosis. There may be an irresistible urge to lie down and go to sleep, and the gait may become unsteady. Double vision, nasal speech, and difficulty in swallowing with hypersalivation and descending paralysis may follow due to the effect of the postsynaptic neurotoxin. Mental confusion, shallow breathing, or actual fighting for breath herald respiratory failure, and the patient may drown in secretions or choke on vomitus unless care is taken to prevent this. Convulsions and coma are followed by death. Krait envenoming is usually painless initially but may later cause violent abdominal pain; such venoms contain presynaptic and/or postsynaptically acting neurotoxins.

Management. The most effective first aid treatment for neurotoxic elapid bites is pressure immobilization, the application of a long crepe (semi-elastic) bandage wound around the bitten limb, starting beyond the site of the bite and extending up to the groin/axilla. This bandage should be applied as tightly as for a sprain. In practice, most bandages are applied too loosely to be effective. With the addition of a splint to ensure immobilization, this method delays absorption of larger molecular weight venom components, such as phospholipase A2 presynaptic neurotoxins, by compressing lymphatics and veins. This may delay the onset of neurotoxicity until the patient reaches hospital.

Careful observation is required to detect early symptoms of systemic envenoming; ptosis must not be mistaken for drowsiness. Anticholinesterases, such as edrophonium and neostigmine, may improve neuromuscular transmission by prolonging the action of the physiological transmitter, acetylcholine. This effect may be dramatic in the case of cobra and death adder bites. A test dose (Tensilon test) is appropriate in all cases of neurotoxic envenoming. Atropine must be given first to block undesirable muscarinic effects of acetylcholine. Neurotoxic envenoming demands that antivenom therapy be administered in the same way and with the same precautions described for treatment of envenoming by vipers.

Progressive neurotoxic envenoming results in life-threatening bulbar and respiratory paralysis. Early endotracheal intubation and assisted ventilation, either manual or by mechanical ventilator, is life-saving and is usually required for only 12 to 48 hours. Certain cobras attack by rearing up and spitting a jet of venom for 1 to 2 meters. If this venom enters the eye, it causes severe pain, blepharospasm, lachrymation, erythema, edema, and visual changes. Provided that the eye is immediately irrigated with water, saline, or in an emergency, with urine, these symptoms abate. If venom is allowed to stay in contact with the cornea, ulceration and secondary panophthalmitis may result. Corneal abrasions can be detected by fluoresein staining or slit lamp examination. Blindness is an important sequel.

Seasnakes

More than 50 species of venomous seasnakes occur in the coastal waters of east Africa, the Persian Gulf, the Arabian Sea, India, Sri Lanka, New Guinea, Australia, the Indian Ocean, and the Pacific Ocean. They have small heads with nostrils opening on the top of the snout, bodies up to 3 meters in length, and flat rudder-like tails. Seasnakes have short, fixed fangs. They occasionally bite bathers; however, the most common victims are fisherman who empty their nets by hand.

Clinical Features

Bites are almost painless, and there is negligible local swelling. However, if sufficient venom has been introduced, systemic envenoming normally becomes evident within 30 to 60 minutes of the bite. The venom causes generalized rhabdomyolysis of striated muscle, producing tender, painful muscles so that movement may be extremely painful. After 3 to 6 hours, the urine becomes dark brown or black due to the presence of myoglobin. Muscle weakness first affects the proximal limb muscles. Neurotoxicity causes ptosis, double vision, weakness of facial and tongue muscles, and eventually, generalized paralysis with respiratory failure. Hyperkalemia, another consequence of rhabdomyolysis, may cause cardiac arrest and is later aggravated by acute renal failure.

Management

The patient must be conveyed to hospital without delay. Absence of myalgia 2 hours after the bite makes serious envenoming less likely, but slower evolutions have been reported. Patients with envenoming require seasnake antivenom, which if given at the first sign of muscle involvement, produces a dramatic recovery within a few days. If renal failure has developed, dialysis is usually required.

Venomous Back-fanged Colubridae

Systemic envenoming by these few species causes bleeding and coagulopathy, complicated by hemolysis and renal failure. Antivenoms are available only against the venom of the African boomslang and against that of *Rhabdophis* species, Yamakagashi and rednecked keelback, in Japan. In the rare event of bites by other back-fanged colubrids, only supportive treatment can be given because there is no response to non-specific antivenoms.

Atractaspididae

Mole Vipers, Burrowing Adders

Atractaspis species, formerly regarded as vipers, are burrowing snakes that have been reported as being responsible for severe envenoming and occasionally deaths. These snakes have long erectile front fangs, which are extended laterally along the side of the upper jaw. Local

effects of the venom include pain, swelling, erythema, and lack of sensation; systemically envenomed patients are sometimes reported to
show signs of cardiotoxicity, with ECG changes, and hypertension as
well as early autopharmocological effects. No antivenom is available for
treating envenoming by these snakes.

Eye Diseases

Blindness, a personal tragedy in any country, is both an individual and
a family disaster in the tropics. When vision is lost, so is the ability to
hunt, farm, and avoid the assaults of animals and the constant threat of
accidents. Blindness is prevalent throughout the tropics; the fact that
most of it is caused either by ignorance or by preventable and treatable
conditions compounds the disaster.

At present, three of the most important causes of blindness in the
tropics are cataract, vitamin A deficiency, and trachoma. Cataract is
much more common in the tropics than in temperate climates, occurs
at an earlier age because of the greater exposure to ultraviolet light,
and the simple surgery required to restore vision is often unavailable.
An estimated 5 million blind people in India and Africa need surgery;
in Nepal, cataract accounts for 84% of avoidable blindness.

Vitamin A Deficiency

This is a serious threat to the sight and even the life of preschool children through much of the tropics. It is estimated that 250,000 children
become blind from this easily preventable disorder each year.

Physiology

Vitamin A, or retinol, is a fat-soluble, unsaturated alcohol found in
animal foods. Liver, milk, and milk products are the best sources of
active retinol. Plants containing carotene pigments also yield retinol;
dark green vegetables, yellow fruits, tomatoes, and carrots are prime
sources. The vitamin is also present in large amounts in red palm oil.
Carotenes are converted into retinol in the small intestinal mucosal
cells; it takes three times more carotene than retinol to supply the
body's needs. Retinol is stored in the Kupffer cells of the liver, released

into hepatocytes and eventually reaches the tissues bound to prealbumin. Normal serum concentrations are 20 to 49 micrograms per 100 ml. Retinol does not cross the placental barrier freely, and newborn infants have very low stores; they must depend upon their mother's milk for an adequate supply.

Retinol is required for the formation of rhodopsin, the photosensitive pigment of the retinal rods needed for night vision. It is also required for the maintenance of the cuboidal epithelium of the bulbar conjunctiva and the surface of the cornea, the only sites where such delicate epithelium is exposed to the environment. The adult requirement for the vitamin is 12 micrograms per kg bw, but young children require three times as much. One international unit (IU) of vitamin A equals to 0.3 microgram of retinol.

Clinical and Pathological Features

Minor manifestations of vitamin A deficiency may be seen at any age. The first sign of deficiency is night blindness. Children may stumble in the evening or grope for objects in the gloom; symptoms tend to come on suddenly and be of limited duration. Examination of the eyes at this time will reveal a loss of the glistening effect of the scleral conjunctiva: xerosis. Dry, lackluster patches develop with thickening and vertical wrinkling; this has been likened to sandbanks at receding tide. There may be a smoky pigmentation covering the conjunctiva. Even more characteristic are Bitot's spots, which are foamy plaques with a greasy surface, usually triangular in shape. They are quite superficial and can be readily removed, revealing a rough under-surface.

The danger of loss of vision exists as soon as the cornea becomes affected by xerosis. The surface of the cornea becomes rough and granular, with a bluish or milky haze. Inflammation and vascularization are minimal. Corneal ulceration may follow, the ulcers being small, peripheral, round, and sharply demarcated. If unchecked, the ulcers extend to Bowman's membrane, and eventual scarring will interfere with vision even after effective vitamin replacement.

The final stage may come on with great suddenness. Keratomalacia is associated with dissolution of the corneal stomal collagen. A large section of the cornea, or the whole of it, may become necrotic, melting into a gelatinous mass. The cornea bulges forward and can perforate, with the inner contents of the eye herniating. The globe is destroyed, and blindness is permanent. Fortunately, one eye tends to be affected before the other so that urgent treatment may save the sight in the other eye.

The most common precipitant of keratomalacia is measles in a vitamin A–deficient child. They develop anorexia, and thereby critically reduce vitamin A intake. Measles itself is associated with a bilateral keratoconjunctivitis. The other common precipitating factor is kwashiorkor, in which the prealbumin-carrying retinol-binding protein is reduced. The diagnosis of severe vitamin A deficiency must be made on clinical grounds; there is no time for confirmatory tests.

The child should be given 200,000 IU of retinol palmitate by mouth or stomach tube plus 100,000 water miscible units administered IM. Corneal ulceration is treated by topical antibiotics, either tetracycline ointment 4 times daily or by antibiotic drops given hourly. One percent atropine ointment is also applied, and either the eyelids are closed by strapping, or an eye pad is applied.

Prevention

The essential public health approach to vitamin A deficiency is persuading parents of the importance of including green vegetables, carrots, and certain fruits in the diet of young children.

They should also be warned that dried, skimmed, unfortified milk is dangerous because it contains no vitamin A. In the absence of carotene-rich foods, breast-feeding should be prolonged. In regions where red palm oil is used for cooking, vitamin A deficiency does not occur. Effective protection can also be obtained by administering 200,000 IU of vitamin A to preschool children every 6 months. It is tasteless and may be given in a small spoon, or delivered from a capsule squeezed on to the tongue of the child. Children with measles or kwashiorkor should routinely be given additional vitamin A.

Trachoma

Trachoma is a chronic follicular keratoconjunctivitis caused by infection with *Chlamydia trachomatis*. This condition is particularly prevalent in the hot, dry, dusty regions of the Middle East, in parts of the Indian subcontinent, and among the aboriginals of Australia.

The Organism
Chlamydia trachomatis is a 350 mm elementary body, originally assumed to be a virus, but now accepted as a bacterium. Like a virus, it grows both in yolk sac cells of chick embryo and on tissue culture. The organism contains both RNA and DNA, and is sensitive to most antibacterial drugs.

Pathology
Trachoma is transmitted from eye to eye on fingers and clothes, or by flies contaminated with infective nasal discharges or tears. The *Chlamydia* multiply in the superficial cells of the upper tarsal surface, producing a mild inflammatory response associated with epithelial proliferation, follicle formation, and papillary hypertrophy. If secondary infection, or reinfection, does not occur, full healing soon follows.

The major lesions of trachoma result from repeated infection, which is associated with developing hypersensitivity. Papillary and follicular hyperplasia, accompanied by an inflammatory infiltrate and pannus formation, spreads to the limbus and upper part of the cornea, producing a punctate keratitis. Continuing infection may lead to corneal ulceration or complete obliteration. Late-stage healing is associated with severe scarring. Conjunctival scars, originally fine, become converted into strong bands or sheets leading to inversion of the eyelid—entropion—causing the eyelashes to impinge on the cornea, producing further keratitis.

Clinical Features
The incubation period is 4 to 12 days. The initial infection is usually mild and often goes unnoticed. There may be increased ocular itching and lachrymation. Eversion of the upper eyelid will reveal yellow or white pinhead-sized, slightly elevated follicles beneath the epithelium. This condition tends to remit spontaneously. Unfortunately, in endemic areas, especially in children, repeated infection is the rule,

and secondary infection is very common. In these circumstances, symptoms are aggravated, and there is often a mucopurulent discharge. The upper tarsal conjunctivae may be covered with thick follicles from which mucoid material may be squeezed out. Dirty gray follicles appear on the limbus, and pannus may be seen extending down over the upper part of the pupil.

With secondary infection, the whole conjunctiva becomes red and velvety, and there may be palpebral edema. Examination of the cornea may reveal an inflammatory infiltrate, punctate keratitis, opacities, and superficial ulceration. The earliest sign of scarring is irregular migration of the openings of the Meibomian glands onto the inner surface of the lids. The eyelashes turn inward and rub on the cornea, leading to edema, ulceration, and scarring, with eventual blindness.

Diagnosis

Trachoma should be suspected in any child in an endemic area with a mucopurulent infection of the eyes lasting more than a few weeks. Confirmatory signs are the characteristic appearances, especially the presence of follicles on the conjunctiva of the upper lid. The diagnosis is confirmed by finding inclusions—Halberstaedter-Prowazek bodies—in conjunctival cells. To obtain a specimen, the conjunctiva is carefully and lightly scraped with a spatula, the cells being spread thinly on a fat-free slide. The preparation is then fixed with alcohol and stained with iodine, Giemsa, or fluorescent antibody.

Treatment

Treatment is with oral tetracycline, the advantages of which outweigh any possible effect on the teeth of children. At the same time, 1% tetracycline ophthalmic ointment or 1% tetracycline eye drops are applied 2 to 4 times daily for 3 weeks, and then repeated at monthly intervals for 6 months. Surgical correction of entropion can be a sight-saving operation.

Acute Hemorrhagic Conjunctivitis

This condition, first recognized in Ghana in 1969, has now spread to much of the tropical world. The infecting organisms are either

Coxsackie virus A 24 or *Enterovirus 70*. After an incubation period of less than 24 hours, there is an acute onset of conjunctival irritation and a profuse watery discharge. There may be photophobia and swelling of the eyelids, and petechiae appear on the bulbar conjunctivae. These may become confluent. Some patients become febrile and develop pre-auricular lymphadenitis and transient corneal opacities. The attack usually lasts 3 to 4 days, but occasionally lasts as long as 10 days. In India and southeast Asia, *Enterovirus 70* conjunctivitis may be followed after a period of 7 to 10 days by neurological complications. These include radiculomyelitis, cranial, and peripheral nerve palsies, and Guillain-Barre syndrome.

Mechanical Factors

The direct effects of wind and dirt in arid areas are largely responsible for the prevalence of pterygium in the tropics. As this corneal growth occludes the pupil, visual loss follows; surgical removal of the pterygium is the only effective therapy.

Glare conjunctivitis is another danger in the bright desert areas of the tropics. The conjunctiva is desquamated by ultraviolet rays, producing an excruciating blindness. Treatment includes topical use of atropine and cocaine and rest in a dark room; antibiotics are often indicated to control secondary infection. Patients who plan to visit the tropics should be advised to bring Polaroid or reflecting sunglasses.

The final, and perhaps the most important cause of eye damage in the tropics, defies exact classification. The roles of ignorance, filth, and neglect in the etiology of tropical blindness are complex; they may be primary causes, and they are, unfortunately, almost always complicating factors. Their elimination will depend—as do almost all advances in tropical medicine—on general improvements in education, social, and personal hygiene, and water distribution, as well as on an expansion of medical and public health facilities and knowledge.

Heart Diseases

Tropical populations develop the same heart disorders as those in temperate climates, but the incidence is often quite different. Ischemic heart disease is relatively rare in the tropics; angina is usually due to syphilitic aortitis; rheumatic heart disease with valvular defects is extremely prevalent in children and adolescents. Pericarditis, due to suppurative organisms, amebiasis, or tuberculosis, is common. Acute cardiomyopathy is much more frequent in the tropics, and is a major cause of obstetrical morbidity and mortality in multiparous women. The tropical cardiac list already considered includes Chagas' disease, pulmonary hypertension in schistosomiasis, and iatrogenic congestive failure due to over-enthusiastic IV treatment of patients with malaria, severe anemia, and malnutrition. Two other important causes of heart failure deserve special mention.

Cardiovascular Beri Beri

The most important manifestations of acute vitamin B1 deficiency are acute heart failure and encephalopathy. Although the latter is now rare, cardiac or "wet beri beri" afflicts young, displaced bachelors eating unbalanced diets; it is also seen in infants. Instant recognition is vitally important because although delay may be fatal, treatment is simple and rewarding.

Pathology
The accumulation of lactic acid, pyruvic acid and other metabolites causes dilatation of vessels, water and sodium retention, and a considerable increase in blood volume. The venous return to the heart is increased beyond its capacity to respond, and cardiac dilatation is followed by a fall in output.

Clinical Features
The first symptoms are usually edema, increasing fatigue, and some degree of breathlessness. There may also be upper abdominal discomfort, pain, and vomiting. On physical examination, there is peripheral swelling and evidence of a high cardiac output. The skin is warm, the pulse rapid and bounding, the jugular veins are distended, and the liver is enlarged and tender.

The apex impulse is displaced, but apart from a third sound and a pulmonary flow murmur, the heart sounds are normal. X-ray shows general cardiac enlargement, but the electrocardiograph is often normal.

This condition is also seen in infants, ages 2 to 5 months, whose mothers are aneurin-deficient. The mother usually observes that the child is restless, cries excessively, is puffy, and passes little urine. The child ceases to feed, and there may be aphonia. On examination, there is severe venous congestion and abdominal distension. Unless treatment is started urgently, sudden death is a common sequel.

Diagnosis
The diagnosis must be made on clinical grounds for treatment must start immediately. Confirmation of the diagnosis is quickly given by the dramatic response to treatment. It is also supported by a low-serum pyruvate and a difference in red cell transketolase activity before and after addition of thiamine.

Treatment
Critically ill patients may be treated with an intravenous dose of 50 to 100 mg of thiamine (25 to 50 mg for infants). This may cause an anaphylactic reaction, and it is preferable to treat stable patients with 25 mg daily (10 to 20 mg for infants) by IM injection for 3 days followed by oral thiamine. The response to treatment is dramatic; within hours, there is massive diuresis, and a rapid resolution of all abnormalities, so that the patient usually walks out of hospital within 1 week.

Endomyocardial Fibrosis

Eosinophilic Tropical Cardiomyopathy
In 1948, a cardiomyopathy was described in Uganda characterized by extreme thickening of the endocardium due to white, fibrous tissue. This condition has also been recognized in Nigeria, India, and South America, and has affected Europeans living in west Africa.

Pathology. This disease is now considered to be a manifestation of the hypereosinophilia syndrome. In individuals with a high eosinophilia, toxic granules are deposited in the superficial endomyocardium and elicit gross scarring that persists long after the eosinophilia has subsided. The fibrosis is restricted to the inflow tracts, but commonly involves the mitral and tricuspid valves. The result is a restrictive cardiomyopathy affecting one or both ventricles.

When the left ventricle is involved, glistening white scar tissue extends from the apex up the posterior wall, often engulfing the papillary muscle and the posterior cusp of the mitral valve. In the right ventricle, the scarring extends up to engulf the tricuspid valve, and much of the ventricular cavity becomes obliterated.

Clinical Features. Both children and adults are affected. Patients with predominant involvement of the left ventricle present with breathlessness on exertion, or on lying down, and a nocturnal cough. The cardiac impulse is rarely prominent. An early systolic, apical murmur is common. X-ray may reveal a large left auricle and endocardial calcification.

When the right ventricle is predominantly involved, patients complain of fatigue and abdominal distension. They may develop moon faces with periorbital edema and proptosis. In children, growth may be stunted; the musculature is poor, and adolescence is retarded. The hands are often cold, and there may be finger clubbing.

The cardiac impulse is very soft, and a third heart sound is usually present. Auricular fibrillation may occur. There is engorgement of the cervical veins, a large liver, and ascites, but peripheral edema may be minimal. X-ray reveals a large right auricle, and an electrocardiograph shows tall P waves.

Diagnosis. If facilities are available, cardiac catheter studies, angiocardiography, and cardiac biopsy are of considerable help in confirming the diagnosis. Europeans with this condition will have a significant eosinophilia.

Treatment. Surgical removal of excess fibrous tissue and valve repair has given satisfactory results, but adequate facilities for cardiac surgery are rarely available in endemic areas.

Effects of Heat

Throughout the tropics, indigenous diet, activity, clothing, and housing assist man's physiological adaptation to high levels of heat and humidity. Because of ignorance or the pressures of organized trips, the modern tourist has altered the old saying that only "mad dogs and Englishmen go out in the noonday sun."

The body's reaction to thermal stress is influenced by the duration of exposure, humidity, air velocity, amount and type of radiant heat, exercise, and clothing, as well as by the dry bulb temperature. Man responds to an effective temperature rise by vasodilatation, increased sweating, and conservation of salt and water by an increased output of antidiuretic hormone and aldosterone. Water loss from sweating can exceed 10 liters per day. In the desert, a person may lose 7% of body weight and 30 g of sodium chloride in a day. Acclimatization to the high effective temperatures of the tropics is partial and gradual. Studies on subjects in the deserts of Arabia and in the stifling mines of South Africa have demonstrated the need for exposure of at least several weeks' duration before the ability to tolerate elevated temperatures is improved.

The average tourist or victim of a local hot spell will have had no chance for physiological adaptation. In fact, probably the most common ailment of Caucasians first visiting the tropics is severe sunburn, secondary to injudicious exposure to the bright sun with inadequate protective clothing and insufficient time to develop a tan.

Reactions to thermal stress may be either minor or major. The former include prickly heat, or thermogenic anhidrosis, and heat cramps. The flow of sweat in the patient with prickly heat is blocked, and swollen glands produce a papular eruption (mammillaria) on the covered parts of the body. The skin is warm and dry, salt depletion is rare, and the major danger is that the condition predisposes to collapse with hyperpyrexia if exposure to heat is continued.

Heat hyperpyrexia, or heatstroke, is the most serious reaction to high effective temperatures. Studies on the etiology and the pathology of this syndrome are complex; it is sufficient for our purposes to understand that those who are most commonly afflicted are the unacclimatized, who have exhausted their sweating mechanism. As the demands for perspiration are not met, the skin becomes warm and dry, the heat regulating centers of the hypothalamus are damaged, and a vicious cycle of hyperpyrexia to 110°F with decreased sweating ensues. The patient may pass through an agitated, violent stage, followed by lassitude, confusion, and coma. If sweating has not resumed within 12 hours, the outcome is invariably fatal. Prognosis is directly correlated with age, degree of hyperpyrexia, duration of symptoms, the presence or the absence of coma, and the rapidity with which treatment is begun. Those who survive usually have had the benefits of prompt and effective therapy; this primarily involves cooling, which may be accomplished by submersion in cool water, water sponging under constant fanning, or the use of air conditioning.

IV chlorpromazine is a valuable addition to mechanical measures because of its thermolytic and sedative properties. Serum electrolytes and urinary chlorides are normal in patients with heatstroke, and fluid replacement should be limited to a slow IV drip of 5% dextrose and saline. The most crucial differential diagnosis in heat hyperpyrexia is cerebral malaria. If there is any question of *P. falciparum* infection in a hyperpyrexic individual, appropriate therapy should be added to the regimen.

Heat exhaustion is the other major reaction to a torrid effective temperature is. This syndrome is due to an excessive loss of sodium chloride through copious sweating and inadequate electrolyte replacement. As extracellular dehydration becomes marked or is corrected only by replacement with water, cardiovascular collapse ensues. The skin is cool and clammy; the blood pressure is reduced; the body temperature is normal or only slightly elevated; and the sensorium is clear. Serum chlorides are diminished, urinary chlorides are absent, blood urea is elevated, and there may be oliguria with marked albuminuria. Treatment is based on rapid replacement of fluids and electrolytes. The first 500 ml of 5% dextrose and saline should be administered in 10 minutes, and the second in 20 minutes. IV fluids should be continued until blood pressure is maintained, and the urinary flow exceeds 2 liters.

Obviously, it is essential to monitor fluid replacement by careful clinical examination in order to avoid overtransfusion. There is no reason to cool patients with heat exhaustion; in fact, moderate warming with blankets is both desirable and comforting to the patient. Persons who are exposed to hot, humid climates should wear loose clothing, imbibe water freely, and maintain an adequate salt intake. This can be accomplished by increasing dietary salt from 10 to 30 grams per day; inclusion of extra salt in fruit drinks is one palatable means. Many types of salt tablets are commercially available.

Bioterrorism

A number of "tropical diseases" covered in this text, or diseases such as smallpox that were considered in earlier editions but are no longer included because they were thought to have been eradicated in global campaigns, are today emerging as the primary biological agents likely to be employed in terrorist attacks.

Biological terrorism is defined as the intentional or threatened use of bacteria, viruses, fungi, or toxins from living organisms to produce death or disease in humans, animals, or plants. Biological agents have been used as weapons of war since ancient times when wells were polluted with corpses, and infected bodies were catapulted over defensive walls in siege operations. In the twentieth century, mankind became more sophisticated—and perverse—learning how to purposefully kill large numbers of civilians with cholera, plague, anthrax, and various toxins.

Even when live agents are not used, the very threat of bioterrorism can paralyze an entire community. In the United States in 2001, after a handful of criminally transmitted anthrax cases were detected, all the major television networks, the Supreme Court, both Houses of Congress, and numerous postal facilities were simultaneously closed. Medical and law enforcement service were almost overwhelmed by the resultant panic and fear.

Many biological agents have been used in terrorist attacks, but the ideal are those that can be effectively suspended for wide spread dissemination. Science has actually made it possible to "weaponize" some biological agents, allowing them to be prepared as fine particles of uniform size with additives that prevent clumping and promote stability. This form can be easily dispersed, as aerosols. Inhalation is an optimal route for the spread of infectious disease because biologicals are usually colorless and odorless; can be carried on the wind; and survive in food, water, or soil.

The ideal aerosol for maximum infectivity has viable organisms of 2 to 3 microns, thereby allowing the particles to reach the alveolar level of inspiration. Larger-size particles are blocked higher up in the respiratory system, causing less disease.

Biological agents have certain advantages as terrorist weapons; they are cheap, relatively easy to produce, and quite easy to disguise behind a "dual use," such as in laboratory research or drug development programs. Very small amounts are needed to contaminate large geographic areas; agents such as anthrax, tularemia, Q fever, and other have been shown to be carried dozens of kilometers by the wind. This makes it possible for terrorists to release deadly agents from safe, remote areas that are distant from, for example, highly protected urban centers.

The most dangerous agents are considered as Category A threats. Bioterrorism attacks differ from other weapons of mass destruction in that they do not cause immediate or easily recognizable clinical conditions. There is almost always an incubation period with biologic infections, whereas nuclear, radiologic, or chemical attacks are evident as soon as the deadly act occurs. The covert introduction of a biologic agent is usually manifest only days or even weeks after release. Patients will have traveled far from where they were infected, and perpetrators escape the scene of the crime easily.

While diagnosis is almost invariably delayed until signs and symptoms of disease manifest days or even weeks after exposure, there are therapeutic and prophylactic measures that can be employed to counter even the most dangerous bioterrorist attacks. For anthrax, an effective vaccine is available for the military and members of law enforcement agencies as well as for critical care and select public health personnel. Treatment with doxycycline or ciprofloxin is also effective both as a treatment for cutaneous anthrax lesions and as a mass prophylaxis for citizens suspected of being exposed.

A vaccine also exists against plague but does not protect against the deadly pneumonic form of the disease. Various antibiotics, as noted earlier, are effective in treating acute plague, but therapy must be initiated early. There is a vaccine against tularemic infections, but it is rarely given to civilian populations because the frequency of side effects outweighs the benefits; numerous antibiotics are effective. Smallpox can be prevented by vaccination given prophylacticly or within three days of exposure, but once again, side effects are sufficiently common that the benefits of mass inoculation campaigns must be balanced against the likelihood of the terrorist threat. There is also the potential to modify smallpox virus, or to use related viruses, such as monkey or camel pox, and thereby make a standard smallpox inoculation campaign useless. There is no specific treatment available for this deadly and disfiguring disease.

Health care providers, especially primary medical and nursing personnel, are at great risk of becoming secondarily infected with the biological agents listed in Table 8. For the viral hemorrhagic fevers, such as Ebola and Marburg disease, for example, strict reverse-isolation techniques are essential if the treating physician does not wish to join the often-fatal course of the patient. Biodetection depends, to some degree, on sophisticated monitoring systems. However, because of the incubation periods, and movement of populations, the primary diagnostic burden in bioterrorist attacks falls on direct health care providers. Education and awareness are the indispensable requirement for diagnosis. In most major urban centers considered as high risk areas in the United States, public health authorities have initiated biosurveillance techniques based on the reporting of unusual patterns of illness seen in hospitals or pharmacies. This "syndromic surveillance" is a critical tool for the future, one based on collecting and interpreting observations of doctors and nurses who may not appreciate, in a single clinical case, a trend that on multiple findings, moves from suspicious to conclusive.

Table 8. Category A Threats

High priority agents that pose a risk to national security
Easily disseminated or transmitted and with high mortality
Major public health impact
Panic and social disruption
Biological Agents
Anthrax (*B. anthracis*)
Botulinum toxin (*C. botulinum toxin*)
Plague (*Y. pestis*)
Smallpox (*V. major*)
Tularemia (*F. tularensis*)
Filoviruses (Ebola, Marburg) Arenaviruses (Lassa)

Advising Tropical Travelers

Many physicians in the developed world will deal with tropical medicine only when asked to help prepare a tourist for a tropical journey. Travel, whether for business or pleasure, has increased tremendously in recent years due to availability, relative ease and low cost. International travel increased from 20 million persons in 1950 to 935 million by 2010, and this trend continues almost exponentially. The World Travel and Tourism Council in London has published figures showing that worldwide business and travel expenditures for 2010 were $3.7 trillion, up from $2.5 trillion in 2000.

More people than ever have the facility, finances, and desire to see new places, new faces, and new things, and to travel in health. There are few, if any, areas of the world where, with adequate preparation and using a common-sense approach, even the most timid cannot wander, adding new dimensions to their routine lives. But it is amazing how liberal tourists are when purchasing air tickets or hotel accommodations, and how foolish they can be in scrimping on a modest investment to ensure good health on their journey. Even minor medical problems can disrupt a trip and result in curtailing a much-anticipated itinerary. Many health problems can be predicted, and often prevented, by simple advance planning. No set of health recommendations can apply to all. The following advice is general. Ideally, it should be tailored to the individual traveler's needs and medical condition.

First, it is important to realize that travel itself causes both psychological and physical stress. A strange and unfamiliar setting, far from the security of home and family, especially in our turbulent world where political and civil unrest is so common, may make all but the most independent person somewhat anxious. Air travel across time zones often results in the well-recognized phenomenon of "jet lag," a disruption of one's 'round-the-clock pacemaker that sets the tempo of waking, sleeping, and other metabolic processes. Some of these stresses are essentially unavoidable and call for simple adaptation. Others can be alleviated or eliminated by a few basic precautions. One should advise the traveler to expect—and not be panicked by—minor changes in diet, climate, or routine; these are usually easily accommodated by the prepared traveler.

Wherever one travels, remember that the tourist will be away from the comfort of knowing that their own doctor and pharmacist are quickly at hand to respond to concerns. In most parts of the world, however, they are never more than a telephone call away, and it is sensible to include these telephone numbers with other essential travel documents. The tourist should obviously discuss a proposed trip with one's own doctor or with a specialist in international health. Certainly, one should do so if suffering from any current or chronic medical condition, regardless of whether it is considered serious or debilitating. A health problem that may not be particularly troublesome under normal circumstances can become a critical challenge because of the mode of travel, the climate, or the geography of the destination, or even the purpose of the trip. There are obvious differences between the advice given to a person who goes to Africa for a day to deliver a single lecture in a capital city and the counsel offered to the tourist going on safari, or backpacking in rural areas, exploring different cultures, lifestyles, and diet.

There are some common challenges. Brand names of medications may be unfamiliar overseas, and many drugs are simply unavailable in developing nations. There may be language and cultural barriers preventing adequate communication with a new physician in a strange land. The panic that often seizes people who become sick abroad is frequently out of all proportion to the illness, but a lack of basic knowledge of one's medical condition, a lack of simple and safe self-remedies, and a lack of preparation often contribute to an overwhelming sense of impending doom. It is advisable to begin medical planning well before a trip to a tropical area, especially in a developing land. If inoculations are required or recommended, it may take several weeks before an effective level of immunity is attained. Frantic last-minute efforts to obtain "shots" are ill advised and further complicate the ordinary stress surrounding an overseas journey.

The traveler should be encouraged to strive for medical self-sufficiency, especially in the tropics where health facilities and approaches may be very different from that which is so easily taken for granted in developed nations. A sick, frightened patient is vulnerable; and one's judgment, far from loved ones, a trusted family physician, or competent specialists, may be faulty. Preventive inoculations, medications, and advice will, hopefully, keep the traveler well enough to avoid unnecessary medical care while away from home. This is not always possible. One can, when absolutely necessary, identify (for example) an English-speaking physician by contacting (if available) one's local Embassy. Telephone advice from home can, obviously, be both helpful and comforting.

On return from abroad, the traveler should be encouraged to seek medical advice if one has been unwell or becomes so within weeks of returning home. It is possible to develop malaria, for example, despite rigorous care and prophylaxis, after returning home. If one has traveled extensively in tropical lands, it is advisable to have a checkup regardless of how one is feeling since many tropical disorders can be diagnosed before any symptoms appear.

A medical kit can be customized to suit each individual. Prescription medications taken on a regular basis should accompany the traveler; one should have a sufficient supply of medication to last the entire trip, plus a buffer in case of loss or unforeseen delay in returning home. All prescription medications should be labeled with the proper drug name (not just the trade name, because these vary from place to place) and the dosage in each tablet or capsule. It is wise to carry essential medications in hand baggage lest lost luggage leave the tourist sick as well as angry. The medical kit should also include such basic first aid items as bandages, thermometer, scissors, medicated powder, aspirin, and even a small supply of toilet tissue, which is a nicety that may well be unavailable on the road.

Those with chronic health problems should consult their own physicians regarding other items that may be needed. An insulin-dependent diabetic, for example, must carry adequate needles and syringes as well as urine-or blood-testing equipment. It may be necessary to have a formal letter stating that syringes are medically necessary; at the very least, syringes should be packed in a medical kit so that they do not appear as casual drug paraphernalia to a suspicious customs official in a foreign land. Diabetics should also carry a nonsugar sweetener when traveling because these are often unavailable in other countries.

It is also essential for anyone suffering from a chronic condition in which crises may occur—such as epilepsy, known allergies of a life-threatening nature, and continuing corticosteroid therapy—to carry a full medical record. Then, in the event of loss of consciousness or severe injury, healthcare personnel overseas can be aware of special needs. For those with heart disease, a recent electrocardiogram, for example, can be very helpful. People who rely on spectacles or contact lens should carry an extra set as well as a prescription.

In addition, the following items may prove useful:

Analgesic tablets—mild painkillers, such as acetaminophen—are important. These medications are effective in relieving common pains associated with muscle or joint strain, sunburn, or headache. For those embarking on a more risky safari or mountain climb, more potent painkillers are an advisable addition to the kit. It is pain that usually forces patients to seek medical care. If pain can be controlled in a remote area, one is more likely to receive superior attention at a central hospital or, even better, at home.

Antihistamine tablets can reduce ear problems due to pressure changes in air travel, especially during takeoff and landing. They also relieve itching due to insect bites and rashes caused by plants. However, one must advise the traveler that these drugs may cause drowsiness and blurred vision. Alcohol should not be taken with these tablets. An antihistamine cream is useful for local application to insect bites.

Antinausea tablets, or transdermal slow release tapes, are good drugs for those who routinely suffer from motion sickness.

Antacids, either in tablet or liquid form, can alleviate abdominal upsets caused by unfamiliar food and drink.

Decongestant tablets provide rapid relief from clogged nasal passages or sinus congestion due to altitude changes or minor colds.

Antidiarrheal agents should accompany anyone traveling to areas offering unaccustomed cuisine. Some degree of gastrointestinal reaction is expected; a slight alteration in bowel habit is generally predictable and may require no remedy except patience. Traveler's diarrhea (TD) is a syndrome characterized by two-fold or greater increase in the frequency of unformed bowel motions. Episodes are generally self-limited and require only simple replacement of fluids and salts lost in diarrheal stools. If severe diarrhea or cramps occur, synthetic antimotility agents can be useful to provide temporary relief. They should not be used longer than 48 hours if the traveler has a high temperature or is passing blood in the stool. In such situations, medical aid should be advised, or self treatment with an antibiotic can be begun. I do not advise routine use of antibiotics to prevent diarrhea. Many such compounds have been in vogue during the past quarter century but have proved either ineffective or dangerous.

Broad-spectrum antibiotics. One cannot carry a pharmacy when traveling, but it is prudent to have a single broad-spectrum antibiotic available, whether for self treating an abscessed tooth, severe bronchitis, gastroenteritis, or a festering foot wound. The physician will obviously advise the tourist regarding the indications for therapy, proper dosage, and possible side effects.

Antimalarial tablets. For those traveling to many parts of Africa, Latin America, southeast Asia, and the Middle East, these are the most important part of the medical kit. This topic is considered in detail in the chapter on malaria.

Inoculations

There has been heartening progress in the worldwide battle against infectious disease in recent years. However, many epidemics still occur, particularly in the developing countries of the tropics and subtropics. The international traveler can be protected against certain diseases by specific inoculations as well as by prophylactic medications. However, it does not necessarily follow that the more inoculations one provides, the healthier the traveler is likely to stay. Inoculations should be selectively administered.

Because international patterns of disease are shifting constantly, one should discuss a planned itinerary with a tropical medicine or travel specialist well in advance of departure. This physician would then administer or prescribe appropriate vaccines or other prophylaxes suited to individual needs.

Inoculations should be recorded on a standard yellow International Inoculation Certificate booklet. Yellow fever and cholera vaccinations must also be stamped by a recognized authority. While yellow fever, plague, and cholera are currently the only internationally notifiable diseases, the World Health Organization (WHO) is in the process of substantially revising these regulations to include other significant global threats, such as avian flu and SARS. The following brief comments cover the most common inoculations in alphabetical order.

Cholera

The risk of cholera to Europeans and Americans traveling to endemic regions is so low that it is doubtful whether this vaccination is of much medical benefit, except for medical personnel working in disaster zones or when it is legally required: for example, in mass situations, such as the annual Hajj for Moslems on a pilgrimage to Mecca. However, there have been major outbreaks of cholera recently in Haiti and Latin America as wel as troubled areas of Africa and Asia. Countries can insist on a valid Cholera Certificate for entry even though WHO no longer endorses this view. One cholera inoculation is sufficient to fulfill requirements, but it lasts for only 6 months.

Hepatitis A

This widespread and highly contagious viral infection is spread by contaminated water or poor hygienic practices in food preparation (p. 273). Immunization had traditionally been provided by administering a passive antibody boost in the form of immune serum globulin given just prior to the date of departure; a 4 cc injection lowers attack rates by about 80% for 3 months. It should also be noted—because it is so often asked about—that gamma globulin is manufactured in such a manner that no living agent, including virus particles, have been demonstrated to survive. Gamma globulin is still utilized when travelers do not have adequate time for the new vaccines to take effect.

Today, the preferred protection is an attenuated viral vaccine (Havrix). Two injections of this vaccine 6 months apart offer long-lasting protection and is the preferred approach. It must be stressed that no inoculation obviates the necessity to take care in what one eats and drinks. A combination Hep A/Hep B vaccine (Twinex) is also available for rapid protection.

Hepatitis B

This virus (p. 143) is transmitted through direct contact with infected blood; this includes sharing needles, unscreened blood transfusion, and sexual contact. Immunization is usually recommended for people who are going to live and work in areas highly endemic with hepatitis B. Three injections are required that for maximum protection, must be spaced over a 6 month period. A full series will protect for many years.

Japanese B Encephalitis

Outbreaks have occured throughout rural southeast Asia, southern India, and even in large cities in Vietnam (p. 141). A series of two inoculations spaced over 2 to 4 weeks offers good protection; this is recommended if one is to travel in such endemic rural areas for more than 3 weeks.

Meningitis

This often-fatal disease is endemic throughout the tropics. The specialist in international health will know where recent outbreaks have been reported and, if one's itinerary indicates exposure, a single multistrain meningitis vaccination is indicated. In recent years, bacterial meningitis has been endemic in northern India and Nepal and widespread throughout west and central Africa and in parts of southeast Asia.

Polio

This paralyzing disease, now extremely rare in the United States or Europe, tragically exists in parts of west and central Africa, and also in the Indian subcontinent. For adults and children who have been previously immunized, a trivalent booster dose is sufficient. Adults who have had no prior vaccination should receive 2 doses, 4 to 8 weeks apart.

Rabies

Travelers to rabies endemic countries should be aware of what action to take in the event of an animal bite (p. 91). Pre-exposure vaccination with human diploid cell rabies vaccine (HDCV) provides protection, and is valuable where there is likely to be sufficient exposure coupled with a probable delay in reaching medical aid. It should be stressed that preexposure immunization does not offer full protection from this fatal infection, and prompt attention is essential after any bite in the tropics.

Tetanus

Most travelers from developed lands will have been previously immunized; a booster dose every 7 to 10 years is necessary. The inoculation for adults can readily be combined with diphtheria and pertussis. There have been major diphtheria outbreaks in Russia and Eastern Europe in recent years.

Tuberculosis

Tuberculosis (p. 85) is not a major hazard for most tourists, but selected travelers anticipating high exposure should have a tuberculin test prior to and after travel.

Typhoid Fever

Typhoid fever is another common and serious bacterial infection with transmission rates related to poor standards of personal hygiene and sanitation. It is prevalent throughout Africa, Asia, and Central America and South America. Setails regarding available inoculations are provided in the section on Bacterial Infections.

Yellow Fever

A completed International Certificate of Vaccination is required by many countries in Africa and Latin America as a condition for entry; this requirement can apply to travelers who merely stop over in a country that is categorized as an endemic area. The inoculation is valid for 10 years. It should not be given to infants younger than 1 year of age, and only to pregnant women if travel to an endemic zone is unavoidable.

Special Considerations

Special consideration in providing immunization is demanded if any of the following points apply. Make sure to ask a patient whether he suffers from, or is affected by, the following topics.

Allergies

Some vaccines contain minute amounts of allergenic substances. Any allergy to any drug—particularly antibiotics—or any food allergies, may be a contraindication.

Altered Immunocompetence

The immune system can be suppressed by disease or drugs. A physician should enquire about any alteration in immunological status before any vaccinations are given. Diseases of particular concern include: leukemia, lymphoma, other forms of cancer, and the acquired immunodeficiency syndrome (HIV/AIDS). Treatment with corticosteroids, chemotherapy for malignant disease, or radiation may also suppress the immune system temporarily.

Febrile Illness

Minor illnesses, such as the common cold, are not an adequate basis for postponing inoculations. However, if there is moderate to severe febrile illness, immunization should be deferred until recovery has occurred.

Pregnancy

If a patient is pregnant, or thinks she might be pregnant, many inoculations can be given if the benefit outweighs hypothetical risks. However, live viral vaccines—such as measles, mumps, rubella, and oral polio—should not be given to pregnant women.

Breast Feeding

There may be problems with some vaccines during breast feeding, and this should be discussed with the mother.

Food and Drink

These are a source of potential grief, as well as great joy, to those who travel. Primarily, but not exclusively, the concern applies to developing countries where modern sanitary facilities are the exception rather than the rule; where sewage disposal, human and animal, is distinctly substandard; where food preparation is rarely handled in a scrupulously hygienic manner; and where climate and insects add further risks to the unwary traveler. As a basic rule, the old adage, "If you cannot boil it, cook it, or peel it, then forget it," should apply. Common sense is the indispensable ingredient for a safe and happy journey and is the basis for advising tourists regarding diet.

Foods prepared well in advance of serving should be avoided; these include cold plates, custards, pastries, and the like. Particularly when improperly refrigerated, such foods are notorious vehicles for a variety of microbes and parasites, which can cause serious gastrointestinal distress.

Vegetables should be freshly cooked and not simply reheated. They should not be eaten raw. Salads should be avoided. Fresh fruits should not be eaten if the skin has been broken, no matter how slight this may appear. Meats should be thoroughly cooked and consumed while still hot. Undercooked beef and pork are both major sources of tapeworm infestation throughout the tropics.

Fish and other seafood can also be a source of trouble due both to toxins and infectious organisms. Raw or smoked fish can carry tapeworms. Oysters and clams taken from sewage-polluted waters and eaten raw or inadequately cooked are proven culprits in hepatitis and cholera outbreaks. Contaminated fish, especially of the grouper family in the Caribbean, have been incriminated as the cause of a sometimes fatal syndrome called "ciguatera poisoning." All fish and seafood should be fresh, and thoroughly cooked.

Milk, milk products, and foods prepared from them should be avoided in areas where the process of pasteurization is unknown or sterility may be in question. Boiling milk is an alternative, or the traveler may carry a supply of powdered milk. Obviously, water used to reconstitute powdered milk must itself be clear of disease. Soft drinks may or may not be safe. One only has to see bottles in some tropical areas being replenished from a syrup and water mixture that is simultaneously serving a large population of flies to appreciate the possible danger. The safest option is imported canned soft drinks. Alcoholic beverages may or may not be safe. Brand-name imported whiskey, gin, vodka, and wine pose no risk except if ice cubes are added. Beer is usually safe. Alcohol tolerance may be influenced by heat, humidity, and altitude as well as stress.

Water is a prime source of gastrointestinal disease especially, but not only, in tropical areas. Water purification tablets do not destroy all infective organisms, and the bitter taste they produce is no guarantee of safety. Water filters certainly can reduce the quantity of infecting organisms but do not eliminate small parasites, bacteria, or viruses. Care should be taken in the very minimal exposure required even for brushing teeth. The freezing of water to produce ice does not destroy all pathogens. To be safe, water should be boiled for several minutes. One should bear in mind that water boils at a lower temperature, the higher the altitude. Bottled water is now widely available in the tropics, but travelers should always unseal the cap themselves; refilling bottles from a nearby stream or tap is a common practice. Dishes and utensils may also serve as a medium for disease communication. A premoistened, foil-packaged hand wipe can be used to protect a diner in a developing land where hot water and soap may not be available.

Exercise

Routine exercise is an essential component in maintaining a healthy body. To enjoy travel fully, one must be as fit as possible and, for some journeys, preliminary physical training is definitely recommended. A holiday that demands vigorous mountain trekking, for example, should not be scheduled without allowing for a period of adaptation to exertion at high altitudes and exposure to cold, wind, and sun. Similar challenges may face those traveling to the tropics where intense heat can change a routine exercise program into potentially fatal acute dehydration and heat stroke.

There are a few basic principles of muscle and vascular tone that are of particular importance to the air passenger. One should avoid staying in a cramped position for long periods. In the confined space of an economy class seat, it is easy to understand how when sitting upright and immobile, with legs at a right angle at both thighs and knees, one can readily develop a circulatory condition in which stasis of blood leads to clots and emboli. It is important to occasionally extend the legs and stretch the muscles even while sitting. Periodically, one should walk in the aisles and try to improve circulation by standing on one's toes or doing a few knee-bends. Airport hallways and lounges are usually excellent sites for long walks while waiting for flights or during layovers.

Motion Sickness

On shipboard, travelers should be made aware that a room near the water line, and as close as possible to midship, will minimize the dizzying effect of rolling ocean waves. Fresh sea air and dietary discretion are also crucial factors in avoiding seasickness. One can prevent the nausea that can ruin an auto journey by sitting as close as possible to the front of the vehicle with one's seat reclined and eyes closed.

Climatic Extremes

Many a tropical holiday has been ruined by the very sun that tourists seek. Just as one would avoid extreme exercise and exposure on a very hot, humid day at home, similar common sense should be applied overseas, from Karachi to Kowloon. One's dress should be attuned to the climate; avoid tightly woven synthetic fibers that do not allow adequate evaporation of perspiration and interfere with free air circulation. Loose, long-sleeved cotton garments are the most suitable dress for the tropics. Protection against the sun with broad brimmed hats is strongly advised.

Vacationers to resort areas often try to cram their dreams of basking, bathing, and beachcombing into impossibly brief visits. Their main reward may well be a severe sunburn; this can be effectively prevented by controlled exposure and/or the judicious use of sunblock preparations.

Medical evidence suggests that a hot and humid atmosphere places a greater strain on the body than a hot but dry climate. It is also well documented that people suffering from heart disease adapt less readily than others, and that excessive physical activity is often a contributing factor in heat exhaustion and heat stroke. Common sense suggests that the traveler take it slow and easy.

Insects

Numerous arthropods are, as detailed in earlier chapters in this text, vectors for many serious diseases in the tropics. Long-sleeved shirts and long pants offer simple and effective barrier protection. Mosquito netting is often advisable. Most camping stores have handy nylon nets, which weigh only a few ounces and require minimal luggage space; tropical tourists should use nets impregnated with pyrethrums. Insect repellents are usually available in local cities. These should be applied around the neck, ankles, and wrists, and frequently reapplied if there is copious perspiration. Mosquitoes are attracted by light, and the experienced tropical traveler quickly learns to check screens, if they exist, or get under a good net if one wants a comfortable night's sleep.

Venereal Diseases

It is important that the sexually active traveler be fully aware that the incidence of gonorrhea and syphilis in many parts of the world exceeds even the near epidemic proportions currently documented in the

United States and Europe. The traveler who contemplates sexual relations with casual acquaintances must obviously consider the alarming prevalence of fatal HIV/AIDS in the tropics. It is sheer folly to have unprotected sex with new partners in most countries, especially in Africa, or with those working in the sex industry in any country.

Common Sense

Ultimately, one returns to the emphasis for the physician advising tropical travelers to stress common sense. Inoculations and medications are not a substitute for scheduling adequate rest periods and appropriate exercise intervals during a journey; for avoiding excesses, whether in activity or alcohol; or for following basic hygienic practices, especially washing hands after using the toilet and before eating. But with common sense and good medical advice, almost all tourists should be able to travel with joy and in good health.

Epilogue
The Evolution of a Tropicalist

I conclude this Jubilee Edition with some personal reflections on my own professional journey in tropical medicine. When the initial chapters of this book were serialized in *The New York State Journal of Medicine*, I was a young physician who had been introduced to tropical infections on a fellowship in Calcutta, India. I was fascinated by the history of epidemic diseases, by the dramatic clinical presentations of tropical infections, and by the diagnostic and therapeutic challenges they pose.

When I arrived in Calcutta, I also fell in love with a way of life. I seem to find romance in settings that others might—quite legitimately—see only as dirty, broken-down wastelands. Surely those negatives existed in Calcutta. But amidst the fetid stenches of Indian urban decay, I recall the strong aroma of exotic spices. I close my eyes and see saffron robes rather than soiled rags. I hear music in the cacophonous sounds of the slums and in the long silence of a city drenched in the humid heat that comes with the monsoon rains.

Fortune continued to bless my nascent career in tropical medicine. At the beginning of the 1960s, due to the ever-expanding war in Vietnam, doctors in the United States were drafted into military service. I was assigned to the US Navy Medical Corps and, blessedly, first allowed to complete a degree at the London School of Hygiene and Tropical Medicine before being sent to The Naval Medical Research Unit—3 in Cairo, Egypt. As the Unit's Head of Epidemiology and Director of Clinical Tropical Medicine, I undertook, over the next few years, field investigations in Sudan, Somalia, Ethiopia, Egypt, and Turkey, and across the Middle East. Once again, I discovered beauty in areas that are most often described as desolate. The arid deserts and harsh bush of Somalia, or the even more difficult, sodden, mosquito-laden swamps of Sudan became my favored places for epidemiologic exploration. In retrospect, however, I was utterly unaware of the direction that my own medical and academic career as a tropicalist would take.

During this period, I became increasingly aware of the extra-medical complex demands one faced in dealing with the trauma of natural and man-made disasters in areas where there were few resources. These developing, often newly independent, nations could barely cope in relatively stable times. In the face of famine, drought, floods and civil wars, these societies—and their very basic health services— quickly collapsed.

Upon my discharge from the Navy in the mid-1960s, I established a career pattern that included daily clinical work, teaching, and continued field research. Since then, I have been Director of the Tropical Disease Center at Lenox Hill Hospital and, for many years, Clinical Professor of Tropical Medicine and Molecular Parasitology at the N.Y.U. Medical School. For 36 years (1969–2006), I was also the Chairman of the Department of Tropical Medicine at The Royal College of Surgeons in Ireland, and have served as the Consultant in Tropical Medicine for the United Nations Health Service and for numerous international corporations and non-governmental organizations (NGOs).

I was able to maintain close contact with the realities of life in the tropics through semi-annual research trips to Somalia, the Sudan, and Nicaragua, and by responding to complex humanitarian crises, particularly in conflict zones, or after devastating national disasters such as earthquakes. This latter work slowly became my primary interest. I gradually changed my focus from individual diagnosis and therapy to the far broader challenges of providing emergency care to refugees and internally displaced persons.

It is at times of great calamity and suffering—in humanitarian crises—where the developed and developing worlds most intimately interact. These occasions, if mismanaged, cause further divisions in an ever more polarized world between the "haves" and the "have-nots." But, if managed correctly, with forethought and planning, with sensitivity and clinical efficiency, then something profoundly good may emerge. There may be no more important arena in which academic standards need to be urgently applied than in the repetitive humanitarian crises that shame our so-called "civilization."

There are obvious, cruel realities in humanitarian fieldwork, and no amount of diplomatic sophistry can dehumanize the horrors of conflict and the waste of innocent lives. These are human beings, not dull statistics, who suffer and die in such situations. In the sad settings of refugee camps where I have worked, mothers and children are the disposable refuse of global insecurity; becoming a child soldier or a sex slave are terribly realistic options for innocent youngsters.

In humanitarian crises, one also struggles with the dark and tangled roots of hatred and the incipient revenge that blossoms in such unrelenting misery. One quickly becomes aware that there are no simple answers in such situations. Solutions, when they can be constructed, draw on many, many disciplines. It is essential to extend the professional standards that prevail in tropical medicine to the less-disciplined field of humanitarian affairs. Disaster management is an evolving science, embracing every stage: from prevention and preparedness, through rapid assessment and cluster assignments, to the final phases of reconstruction and development.

When I was young, and innocent, I thought I was inordinately important as a medical doctor in a refugee camp. But it did not take long to look around and realize, with growing humility, that those in charge of water or food or shelter or security or sanitation or education were essential partners. It did not take long to realize that no one could accomplish very much working alone. I came to realize that if there were to be any progress in restoring a semblance of stability for those who had lost almost everything, we had to overcome our own restrictive professional barriers.

One had to develop a radically different perspective regarding those treasured academic distinctions we had been taught were so important during medical training. One also had to learn not to be afraid to venture afield as circumstances demanded. Diplomas and degrees can easily become artificial boxes that prevent flexibility. In providing humanitarian assistance, flexibility is an indispensable and absolute necessity.

Rigid definitions of duty cripple programs in the field. There is that inevitable time when, at least in my experience, one must move beyond the traditional confines of any discipline. There had been no courses—except possibly in philosophy, anthropology, or comparative literature—that prepared me for the almost bizarre demands one faces in attempting to establish and manage camps for tens, and sometimes hundreds, of thousands of frightened, ill and endangered people, the vast majority being extremely vulnerable women and children. Three examples demonstrate different challenges that expanded my traditional role as a physician.

Early in my career, I found myself in Southern Sudan, responsible not only for health concerns, but also for providing other basic human services, including security. It certainly was of little help to a young girl to tell her that her malaria was cured if she was raped every time she went foraging for firewood.

In 1972, an earthquake destroyed Managua, Nicaragua. I served as chief medical adviser, sharing a tent with the then President. There, I learned how politics and corruption can pollute so-called "relief missions." A significant percentage of the international aid was openly looted by the President's cronies, and donors did not even complain for "diplomatic" reasons. One sadly realized the limitations of altruism in the face of evil.

Retraining and resettling large numbers of refugees was essential in Somalia after the Sahel drought caused a mass migration across Africa. I was directing camps with almost 1 million refugees, and the only outlet was the Indian Ocean. Trying to teach nomads to abandon an age-old dependency on camels and cattle to seek survival as fishermen was an interesting exercise for an evolving tropicalist. The experiment worked, at least for a while.

There were also obvious diplomatic possibilities in our tropical public health work, and these could—and needed to be—exploited. Medicine offered an almost ideal platform for preventive diplomacy. Almost 50 years ago, in the midst of a raging civil war in Southern Sudan, "corridors of tranquility"—so-called "immunization breaks"—were established. These were *de facto* ceasefire zones, and eventually became temporary bridges to understanding and peace. That peace didn't last, but the effectiveness of those "corridors" is still recalled today by those who struggle to find the elusive common ground in the blood soaked sands of Sudan.

My responsibilities in this field inevitably grew, particularly in the chaotic reality that is far too often, the norm around the globe, especially in conflict prone zones where poverty and aggression prevail. One had to devise new, imaginative, and innovative paths forward. Managing complex humanitarian emergencies, particularly in the midst of conflicts and disasters, is not a field for amateurs. Good intentions are a common, but tragically inadequate, substitute for well-planned, efficiently coordinated, and carefully implemented operations that must have a beginning, a middle, and an end. Compassion and charity are only elements in humanitarian assistance programs; alone, they are self-indulgent emotions that for a short time may satisfy the donor, but will always fail to help victims in dire straits.

When I first began working in complex humanitarian crises, there were almost no standards of training. In fact, there was not even a common vocabulary. What was desperately needed was the creation of a new profession, one that could embrace the many areas of expertise required to provide an overall response. This is where academia had to enter the picture. More than 20 years ago, new, practical, university-level programs geared to the unique needs of international aid workers were developed. At Fordham University in New York, we have, as this book goes to press, more than 1,600 graduates from 133 nations, and one can earn a post-graduate Masters degree, or pursue an undergraduate Minor in this field.

It is primarily in the university where knowledge is analyzed and defined, where good—and bad—practices are studied, where the lessons of the past are distilled in a continuing search for wisdom and understanding. Humanitarian assistance is an ideal area for academic interest. It presents a multidisciplinary challenge, drawing on, among others, the fields of public health and medicine, law and politics, logistics and security, technology and anthropology: indeed, all social, physical, moral, economic, and philosophic arts and sciences.

The multiple causes of, and difficult solutions to, humanitarian crises require an arena for the free, unfettered exchange of ideas where the development of new approaches to overcome the failed *status quo* is encouraged. That is the essential environment of a good university. The university should be—and usually is—the last bastion where open discussions, and respect for differing ideas, prevail. It is society's ultimate refuge from bias and prejudice, and these are among the most significant causative factors in humanitarian crises. The search for answers cannot be limited to the medical school, or the law school, or any other specialized school. It involves all the many, linking disciplines that are the foundation of a true university.

In trying to establish the broadest possible base for programs in humanitarian assistance, much depends on how one approaches problems, and troubled areas. One of the most important lessons of India that has remained with me for life, and has helped determine what I have tried to do and how, was the realization that one must stay calm and focused in the midst of chaos if one wants to help others. There was no time for self-indulgent, personal concerns. The petty needs that so often dominate our lives distract us from getting critical tasks accomplished. One quickly realized, with embarrassment, that our own individual cares simply did not matter much in the face of what others were suffering every day, all day, in the disaster that life offered them.

Since then, during a very full, joyous career—if that is an appropriate description for a journey where there were few guideposts along the way—I've worked in 65 countries, mostly in refugee camps and war zones. I have seen plenty of tragedy during those travels. Many scenes are still seared into my soul: the appalling waste of life and human dignity; pain that I was often unable to relieve; the stares of starving children and the dying gasps of too many mothers after childbirth. Yet I have always realized how privileged I have been to serve, to share, and even begin to identify with those caught in the crossfire of conflicts not of their making. A spiritual solidarity develops in just being with them. They are my brothers and sisters.

But that was not enough. I had to construct solutions to problems that, at least for me, were without precedent. I soon came to understand that tradition and culture were as essential as aspirin or bandages in running a basic medical program. One quickly realized that prejudice and economic exploitation, pride and politics, racism and religion, weather and witchcraft, corruption and incompetence, were all integral parts of the problems one had to address. It is necessary to appreciate the cry of the oppressed, and the burden of ignorance, fear and poverty, if one is to practice medicine in a developing land, especially during—and after—periods of disaster.

In the most sordid situations, I have always felt inordinately humbled to see, often with amazement, but always with admiration, the courage and resiliency of the downtrodden, those who seem to have been totally overwhelmed, but then, like the Phoenix, rise again from the ashes. I have always returned—although part of me never returned—from refugee camps grateful to be allowed to participate in their valiant efforts.

I have helped, even healed, many desperate victims in humanitarian crises, but they in turn, helped, healed, instructed, and changed me. I have been the recipient of their kindness: They who had so little gave their meager supplies to me, and, on more than one occasion, offered to protect me with their lives. I learned much about the values of clan loyalty and family love around campfires in the deserts of Somalia and Sudan, with elders who were guided by values as noble as my Judeo-Christian traditions.

I have been caught behind the lines in armed conflicts, and seen senseless slaughter from Beirut to Managua, and all across the scarred landscape of modern Africa. Somehow in the twisted wreckage of war, and in the squalor of refugee camps, the incredible beauty of humanity prevailed for me, as it does for most of those privileged to work in humanitarian assistance. It is that perspective that sustains us on what otherwise may seem like a journey through hell on earth. It takes time to refocus the romance of youth into reflective, lasting programs in humanitarian crises, to change the passion of love into healing projects. One learned from errors and failures, and then struggled ahead, with more hard work. As Samuel Beckett once wrote, we must "Try again. Fail again. Fail better."

It would certainly have been easier—and safer—to reap the rewards assured by a predictable medical practice at home. However, that was not what fate offered. My wife and I discovered a new world—and ourselves—in politically volatile areas where change and revolution were in the air, and on the streets. Medicine allowed unusual access, even for a Western stranger, in closed, often hostile, societies. We were able to share in the dreams and aspirations of men and women in the developing world who were fighting for freedom, equality, basic human rights, and often their very survival.

The discipline of tropical medicine has taken me in uncharted directions with multiple crisscrossing yet mutually supportive paths: from the isolation of a research laboratory through the examining room and the lecture hall, to epidemiologic field work in remote areas, and to the rough and tumble of refugee camps. This Jubilee Edition draws on all these experiences.

There is no substitute in a medical career for the legitimacy and credibility earned in the daily care of individual patients. This book provides the technical basis for that critical continuity of clinical service. But revisions and additions in successive editions of this text clearly reflect a personal commitment to developing a new, and fully recognized, profession of international humanitarian assistance. My concluding hope for this book is that it may also offer a foundation for those who dare to broaden the horizon of our own discipline and strive in new—yet unknown—ways to help the poor and oppressed masses in the tropics realize a safer, more just and healthy world.

References

Books

Manson's Tropical Diseases, Cooke, G. and Zumla, A., eds., 21st Eed. Saunders, 2009.

Oxford Handbook of Tropical Medicine, Eddleston, M., Davidson, R., et al., 3rd ed. Oxford University Press. 2008.

Basics of International Humanitarian Missions, Cahill, K. M.D., ed. Fordham University Press, 2003.

A Colour Atlas of Tropical Medicine & Parasitology. Peters, W. and Pasoval, G., 5th ed., Mosby-Wolfe. 2003.

Emergency Relief Operations, Cahill, K., M.D., ed. Fordham University Press, 2003.

Short Textbook of Public Health for the Tropics, Gilles, H. M. and Lucas, A., 4th ed., Hodder Arnold. 2002.

Journals

American Journal of Tropical Medicine & Hygiene
Annals of Tropical Medicine & Parasitology
Journal of The Royal Society of Tropical Medicine & Hygiene
Tropical Disease Bulletin

Even in the most remote field locations, the Internet is commonly available, and regular reviews of current management for frequently encountered problems are important. The websites of the following organizations will provide up-to-date guidelines for the management of most tropical diseases, for the Integrated Management of Childhood Illness (IMCI) and the Community Management of Acute Malnutrition (CMAM), and for travelers' health (including vaccinations and malaria prophylaxis).

Other available resources, such as PubMed and Google Scholar, allow rapid review of the latest publications. There are also sites that aggregate sources of information from communities and user generated content. Reliefweb (www.reliefweb.com) is run by the United Nations Office for the Coordination of Humanitarian Affairs (OCHA) and contains links to a wealth of regionally specific information.

Websites

CDC: www.cdc.gov
CIHC: www.cihc.org
GFATM: www.theglobalfund.org
UNAIDS: www.unaids.org
UNHCR: www.unhcr.org
UNICEF: www.unicef.org
UNWTO: www.unwto.org
WHO: www.who.int

Index

The Center for International Humanitarian Cooperation and The Institute for International Humanitarian Affairs

The Center for International Health and Cooperation (CIHC) is a public charity founded by a small group of international diplomats and physicians who believe that health and other humanitarian endeavors sometimes provide the only common ground for initiating dialogue, understanding, and cooperation among people and nations shattered by war, civil conflicts, and ethnic violence. The Center has sponsored symposia and published books, including *Silent Witnesses*, *A Directory of Somali Professionals*, and *Clearing the Fields: Solutions to the Global Land Mine Crisis*, as well as the International Humanitarian Book Series of Fordham University Press listed at the end of this book. This textbook is an essential part of the foundation of the CIHC philosophy.

The Center and its Directors have been deeply involved in trying to alleviate the wounds of war in many areas. A CIHC amputee center in northern Somalia was developed as a model for a simple, rapid, and inexpensive program that could be replicated in other war zones. In the former Yugoslavia, the CIHC was active in prisoner and hostage release and in legal assistance for human and political rights violations, and facilitated discussions between combatants.

The Center directs the International Diploma in Humanitarian Assistance (IDHA) in partnership with Fordham University in New York and the Royal College of Surgeons in Ireland. It has graduated more than 1,500 leaders in the humanitarian world from 133 nations, representing all agencies of the United Nations and major nongovernmental organizations (NGOs) around the world.

The academic arm of the Center, the Institute of International Humanitarian Affairs (IIHA) at Fordham University in New York, offers a graduate Masters Degree in Humanitarian Affairs and an undergraduate Minor program. The CIHC also offers specialized training courses for humanitarian negotiators, international human rights lawyers, and mental health workers in war zones, and now offers a holistic Masters in International Humanitarian Affairs (MIHA) degree program. To learn more about the MIHA, please visit http://www.ford ham.edu/iiha.

The Center has provided staff support in recent years in crisis management in Iraq, East Timor, Aceh, Kosovo, Palestine, Albania, Lebanon, Pakistan, and other trouble spots. The Center has been afforded full consultative status at the United Nations. In the United States, it is a fully approved public charity. The Directors of the CIHC serve as the Advisory Board of the IIHA. The President of the CIHC is the University Professor and Director of the Institute, the CIHC Humanitarian Programs Director is Visiting Professor at the IIHA, and another CIHC Director is the Diplomat in Residence at Fordham University.

Directors

Kevin M. Cahill, M.D., *President*
David Owen, *Secretary*
Boutros Boutros-Ghali
Tim Cross
Francis Deng
Richard Goldstone
Helen Hamlyn
Peter Hansen
Eoin O'Brien, M.D.
Joseph A. O'Hare, S.J.
Peter Tarnoff

About the Author

KEVIN M. CAHILL, M.D., was Professor and Chairman of the Department of International Health and Tropical Medicine at The Royal College of Surgeons in Ireland from 1969 through 2005; the College then created a new Chair in International Humanitarian Affairs, which he currently holds. He is also Clinical Professor of Tropical Medicine and Molecular Parasitology at New York University Medical School and Director of the Tropical Disease Center at Lenox Hill Hospital in New York. He is the University Professor of International Humanitarian Affairs at Fordham University and the President of the Center for International Humanitarian Cooperation.

Professor Cahill has served as Chief Adviser on Humanitarian and Public Health issues to successive Presidents of the United Nations General Assembly. He is a Consultant to the United Nations Health Service, and to numerous foreign governments. He is Chief Medical Adviser for Counterterrorism in the New York Police Department. He is the author or editor of more than 30 books on tropical diseases, humanitarian assistance, and diplomatic and historical topics. He has received dozens of honorary doctorates and diplomatic as well as scientific awards for his work in the tropics.